COPING WITH CHRONIC ILLNESS

PHYSICAL MEDICINE AND REHABILITATION

Additional books and e-books in this series can be found on Nova's website under the Series tab.

PHYSICAL MEDICINE AND REHABILITATION

COPING WITH CHRONIC ILLNESS

MEGHAN MENDOZA
EDITOR

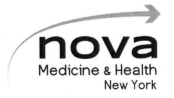

Medicine & Health
New York

Copyright © 2020 by Nova Science Publishers, Inc.

All rights reserved. No part of this book may be reproduced, stored in a retrieval system or transmitted in any form or by any means: electronic, electrostatic, magnetic, tape, mechanical photocopying, recording or otherwise without the written permission of the Publisher.

We have partnered with Copyright Clearance Center to make it easy for you to obtain permissions to reuse content from this publication. Simply navigate to this publication's page on Nova's website and locate the "Get Permission" button below the title description. This button is linked directly to the title's permission page on copyright.com. Alternatively, you can visit copyright.com and search by title, ISBN, or ISSN.

For further questions about using the service on copyright.com, please contact:
Copyright Clearance Center
Phone: +1-(978) 750-8400   Fax: +1-(978) 750-4470   E-mail: info@copyright.com.

NOTICE TO THE READER

The Publisher has taken reasonable care in the preparation of this book, but makes no expressed or implied warranty of any kind and assumes no responsibility for any errors or omissions. No liability is assumed for incidental or consequential damages in connection with or arising out of information contained in this book. The Publisher shall not be liable for any special, consequential, or exemplary damages resulting, in whole or in part, from the readers' use of, or reliance upon, this material. Any parts of this book based on government reports are so indicated and copyright is claimed for those parts to the extent applicable to compilations of such works.

Independent verification should be sought for any data, advice or recommendations contained in this book. In addition, no responsibility is assumed by the Publisher for any injury and/or damage to persons or property arising from any methods, products, instructions, ideas or otherwise contained in this publication.

This publication is designed to provide accurate and authoritative information with regard to the subject matter covered herein. It is sold with the clear understanding that the Publisher is not engaged in rendering legal or any other professional services. If legal or any other expert assistance is required, the services of a competent person should be sought. FROM A DECLARATION OF PARTICIPANTS JOINTLY ADOPTED BY A COMMITTEE OF THE AMERICAN BAR ASSOCIATION AND A COMMITTEE OF PUBLISHERS.

Additional color graphics may be available in the e-book version of this book.

Library of Congress Cataloging-in-Publication Data

ISBN: 978-1-53616-775-7

Published by Nova Science Publishers, Inc. † New York

CONTENTS

PREFACE

The opening chapter *Coping with Chronic Illness* takes into account the impact of the diagnosis on the family, both at the time of the communication of the diagnosis, and in the moment of chronicity, the relationships and of the social context, the coping strategies and the representation of the disease.

Pain management is a growing concern in pediatric cancer patients as pain can originate from multiple sources and negatively influence long-term children well-being. To gain a better understanding of the pain adjustment processes occurring in young patients, the authors analyze a cohort of 30 children and early adolescents with acute leukemia or lymphoma facing cancer-related pain, focusing on the various coping strategies at different stages of therapy.

Additionally, the authors discuss strategies for encouraging family coping efforts and resilience. Future research needs to continue to focus on helping children cope with stress and worry related to their conditions and medical procedures.

Following this, the collection reviews and analyzes the relationship among sociodemographic and clinical variables, psychological morbidity, self-efficacy for coping, illness perceptions and QoL according to disease stages.

The penultimate chapter describes the experience of "continuous" management of adult diabetes at the ASST Spedali Civili of Brescia.

Clinical work has confirmed that an integrated approach focused on the recognition of emotions and relational support is a fundamental element in the management of chronicity.

The concluding paper explores options for chronic illness management in aged care facilities while highlighting the need for more effective illness prevention and positive lifestyle management programmes in the earlier years of life.

Chapter 1 - Among the chronic diseases, Type I Diabetes Mellitus in the middle childhood deserves careful consideration, due to its peculiar characteristics. The first reason is the increase in the incidence of the disease: this increase is constant and real, not due to the simple increase in the number of diagnoses (as in the case of other chronic diseases). Secondly, this disease requires daily and complicated management, which involves not only glycemic controls and insulin administration but also continuous and accurate monitoring of nutrition and physical activity. Finally, middle childhood represents an age group that is somehow neglected by literature, but also interesting for the socio-cultural changes that go through it. The chapter takes into account the impact of the diagnosis on the family, both at the time of the communication of the diagnosis, and in the moment of chronicity, the relationships and of the social context, the coping strategies and the representation of the disease. The authors therefore focused on middle childhood, including data from a pilot study, whose goal is to evaluate the representation of life experience with Diabetes or with a diabetic child, happiness, satisfaction, and adherence to therapy. 50 families (father, patient, mother), with children aged between 8 and 15 years and diagnosed with Type I Diabetes Mellitus for at least three years, were asked to write down their life experience and compile Satisfaction With Life Scale (SWLS Diener, Emmons, Larsen and Griffin, 1984) and the Subjective Happiness Scale (SHS Lyubomirsky, Lepper 1999). Disease management was assessed with Self Care Inventory (SCI La Greca 2004) and with glycated hemoglobin (HbA1c) values. Detailed analyses are reported in the chapter and the results are discussed. In short, the lives of patients with Type 1 Diabetes Mellitus and their parents is certainly demanding, but the disease does not prevent subjective happiness or life satisfaction. The subjects of our example show that they know how to tell their own story, so that they can think and contain it in their mind and maybe that's why they live well, despite the difficulties.

Chapter 2 - Pain management is a growing concern in pediatric cancer patients as pain can originate from multiple sources and negatively influence long-term children well-being. To gain a better understanding of the pain adjustment processes occurring in these young patients, here the authors have analyzed a cohort of 30 children and early adolescents with acute leukemia or lymphoma facing cancer-related pain, focusing on the various coping strategies at different stages of therapy. Specifically, through a mix-method approach integrating quantitative and qualitative data, the authors have characterized a number of coping profiles, internalizing/externalizing symptoms and adjustment difficulties specific for children experiencing cancer-related pain. Altogether, these findings provide a framework with which to predict children at risk of developing maladjustments, in dare need of parent-focused psychosocial interventions.

Chapter 3 - Due to medical advances, more children with chronic illnesses are facing medical procedures. Many of them need assistance learning to cope with medical procedures and extended hospital stays. This chapter provides information on anxiety and worry management strategies for children with chronic illnesses. An emphasis on developing strategies based on the child's existing coping strategies can ensure that strategies will be used in stressful situations and during hospital procedures. Moreover, children with chronic illnesses may be resilient and find hope in many things, so positive aspects of child coping will be presented in this chapter. Additionally, conceptualizing coping as a family affair can be critical to ensuring that the child receives the support he or she needs. Siblings can be critical supports if the child faces an extended hospital stay and siblings are able to stay nearby. Ensuring that the family is coping well, can translate to improved coping for the child and the parent who is with the child, if an extended hospital stay is needed. Children with chronic illnesses and their families may be marked by resilience and a search for meaning and positive functioning as they strive to cope with a difficult family stressor. Thus, strategies for encouraging family coping efforts and resilience also will be a focus of discussion in this chapter. Future research needs to continue to focus on helping the child cope with stress and worry, related to their conditions and medical procedures. At the same time, recording instances of hope and resilience provides a strengths-based approach that can guide ideas for improving family coping and, ultimately, child coping.

Chapter 4 - Breast cancer is the most common malignant tumor in women. Chemotherapy is an adjuvant systemic therapy often used as a treatment for breast cancer with a significant impact on reducing the risk of relapse and overall mortality but with adverse effects on the emotional and functional domains of the patient's life. Women present greater psychological morbidity, higher levels of stress revealed by deregulated cortisol patterns, which are associated with a worse prognosis and tumor growth, less efficient coping strategies and more negative illness perceptions. This chapter reviews and analyzes the relationship among sociodemographic and clinical variables, psychological morbidity, self-efficacy for coping, illness perceptions and quality of life taking into consideration disease stage. The results showed that coping was positively associated with quality of life. Disease stage, treatment side effects, anxiety, depression, illness perceptions and cortisol awakening response (CAR) correlated negatively with QoL. The results suggest that these variables should be considered from the beginning of chemotherapy in interventions and individualized programs adapted to the psychological needs of these patients.

Chapter 5 - For sometimes, the principles of therapeutic education have been applied to treat adult patients with diabetes. Numerous studies have been conducted in this field, but few have monitored the adherence over time (in "chronicity") of operators and patients. Although patients are trained in the management of the disease through therapeutic education, over the years the burden of chronicity often hinders the application of principles, skills and known behaviors. It is therefore necessary to monitor coping strategies, the relational dynamics of patients and family members and in particular the management of emotions and resistance to the management of insulin therapy. Furthermore, it is necessary to listen to their emotional and psychological fatigue and anxiety and offer effective help and support strategies. The same is true for health workers, who also suffer from the burden of chronicity. After reflecting on chronicity, coping strategies, goals of therapeutic education and limits in its implementation, this chapter describes the experience of "continuous" management of adult diabetes at the ASST Spedali Civili of Brescia. The paths dedicated to diabetic patients pay particular attention to the educational-experiential path of Mindfulness, which represents an alternative and appreciated approach based on the recognition of emotions, which is the first filter for their effective management and effective self-care behavior. The results of this pilot study, through the application of BDI, PAID-5 and SCL 90, are disclosed here. Regarding the management of chronicity by the health team, training and supervision groups have been implemented. In particular, data related to 69 supervisions, 43 medical interviews and 23 nurses based on communication skills and competencies were presented and evaluated. Clinical work has confirmed that an integrated approach, focused on the recognition of emotions and relational support is a fundamental element in the management of chronicity.

Chapter 6 - A generation ago health care reformers in Australia became interested in managing care for people with chronic conditions to avoid unnecessary hospitalisation for preventable conditions such as diabetes and cardiovascular disease. Indeed, the national coordinated care trials of the late nineties were predicated on these principles and led to the introduction of new primary care management and funding arrangements for Australia, new Medical Benefits Schedule (MBS) item numbers for health assessments, care planning and care coordination along with strategies to train and support the health workforce. It is now 25 years later, and in the author's retirement work the author is confronted by the enormity of the emerging problem of how to provide good quality, affordable care and stimulation for an expanding population of older and increasingly dependent people with chronic and complex health needs. This led the author to reflect on earlier research work that focused on healthy and productive ageing, care coordination, preventative healthcare and chronic illness management and self-management as strategies for improving health status and reducing hospital admissions for this group of patients. At the same time, we are regularly reminded of the pressing burden of preventable illness in our younger populations along with our failure as a nation to do anything constructive about reducing obesity and morbidity rates in these groups; the main cause of chronic illness in later life. Whilst we have learnt to manage chronic and complex morbidity better due to the immediate pressures that these illnesses are placing on our acute facilities, we are still not addressing adequately the problem of preventable, lifestyle related illness and morbidity and the lack of health literacy in our community that is adding un-necessary and avoidable pressures to our health care funding and service provision systems. As our ageing population in Australia is living longer, but with more complex needs, our younger populations are also being impacted prematurely by complex, but essentially preventable health conditions flowing from poor diet, sedentary behaviours and other lifestyle factors. This paper explores options for chronic illness management in aged care facilities while highlighting the need for more effective illness prevention and positive lifestyle management programmes in the earlier years of life.

In: Coping with Chronic Illness
Editor: Meghan Mendoza

ISBN: 978-1-53616-775-7
© 2020 Nova Science Publishers, Inc.

Chapter 1

COPING WITH CHRONIC ILLNESS: TYPE I DIABETES. A PILOT STUDY IN MIDDLE CHILDHOOD

Paola Manfredi[*] and Cristina Battaglini

Clinical Psychology, Department of Clinical and Experimental Sciences, University of Brescia, Italy

ABSTRACT

Among the chronic diseases, Type I Diabetes Mellitus in the middle childhood deserves careful consideration, due to its peculiar characteristics. The first reason is the increase in the incidence of the disease: this increase is constant and real, not due to the simple increase in the number of diagnoses (as in the case of other chronic diseases). Secondly, this disease requires daily and complicated management, which involves not only glycemic controls and insulin administration but also continuous and accurate monitoring of nutrition and physical activity. Finally, middle childhood represents an age group that is somehow neglected by literature, but also interesting for the socio-cultural changes that go through it.

[*] Corresponding Author's E-mail: paola.manfredi@unibs.it.

The chapter takes into account the impact of the diagnosis on the family, both at the time of the communication of the diagnosis, and in the moment of chronicity, the relationships and of the social context, the coping strategies and the representation of the disease. We therefore focused on middle childhood, including data from a pilot study, whose goal is to evaluate the representation of life experience with Diabetes or with a diabetic child, happiness, satisfaction, and adherence to therapy. 50 families (father, patient, mother), with children aged between 8 and 15 years and diagnosed with Type I Diabetes Mellitus for at least three years, were asked to write down their life experience and compile Satisfaction With Life Scale (SWLS Diener, Emmons, Larsen and Griffin, 1984) and the Subjective Happiness Scale (SHS Lyubomirsky, Lepper 1999). Disease management was assessed with Self Care Inventory (SCI La Greca 2004) and with glycated hemoglobin (HbA1c) values. Detailed analyses are reported in the chapter and the results are discussed. In short, the lives of patients with Type 1 Diabetes Mellitus and their parents is certainly demanding, but the disease does not prevent subjective happiness or life satisfaction. The subjects of our example show that they know how to tell their own story, so that they can think and contain it in their mind and maybe that's why they live well, despite the difficulties.

Keywords: type I diabetes, middle childhood, happiness, satisfaction, coping, narrative, relationships, chronic illness, communication, diagnosis, representations.

1. INTRODUCTION

In line with the trend of all chronic diseases, the incidence of Type 1 Diabetes Mellitus is also increasing. Data from the Diabetology Clinic of the ASST Spedali Civili of Brescia show, from 2014 to date, an increase in incidence of 4% per year. It is important to note that this is a real increase, not attributable to more specific diagnostic capabilities, since often the onset symptom of the disease is now, as in the past, diabetic ketoacidosis.

Beyond the more or less dramatic onset of the disease, an important element in taking care of patients and their families is precisely the communication of the diagnosis. The key critical element is the discrepancy between the expectation of recovery and the chronic scenario.

I.e., after the release of his son and a diagnostic hospitalization, a mother said: "When I brought my child home from the hospital it seemed as if I was bringing him home for the first time, as when just born I brought him home from the nursery".

We can imagine that since childbirth represents a hiatus, similarly the diagnosis of chronic disease also marks a before and an after, which contributes to redefine relevant elements of personal identity (of the patient) and parental functions. Just like the birth of a child, the question that arises regards the skills needed to properly take care of a child. Not only is there, albeit absolutely important, an issue related to the relational and affective dimensions, but there is also a "technical" question since Diabetes Mellitus is considered one of the most demanding diseases from a psychological and behavioral standpoint, being 95% of its management entrusted to the patient.

"Taking care" of your child with Diabetes should have the characteristics of "keeping an eye on": being vigilant, attentive, always keeping in mind, being available, even if you are not always present.[*]

Different competencies and capacities contribute to this objective, of children, parents, family and the relational, health and environmental context. For example, flexibility, the ability to understand requests and resources, which change over time, positive parent-child and family relationships, low levels of anxiety and depression, good resilience, adequate understanding, a good alliance with the health care team, etc. are required (Dukes et al. 2008, Mackey et al. 2011, Monaghan et al. 2012).

In this chapter, we have focused on some topics and contributions in literature, with particular regard to the impact of a family diagnosis, possible symptomatic repercussions, but also to protective factors, such as family cohesion and coping. We have also focused our interest on a developmental age normally scarcely considered in literature: middle childhood, also proposing the data of one of our pilot studies. It is an observational study that analyzes the narratives regarding the illness of the

---

[*] This same attitude should find confirmation and support in the health care team, informed / in the sense shaped by the principles of therapeutic education. As in the image of the matryoshka the little patient must be contained by the family and both, in different and congruent ways, by the team.

patient and his parents, the subjective assessments related to happiness and satisfaction of his own life and Diabetes management.

Unlike previous works on the psychic dynamics of Diabetes Type 1, in which most of the related "negative" aspects were analyzed, our contribution, while taking into consideration disease control and adherence, focuses on the sense of well-being of the patient and his family, despite the daily difficulties due to the illness.

We believe that considering the sense of happiness and satisfaction of the patient and his parents can be an interesting starting point for the development of future research and for building effective relationships with patients and their families. This attention can in fact convey, implicitly or explicitly, significant messages: firstly, that chronic illness is not incompatible with happiness (Manfredi 2017) and that there is a positive attitude in health workers; we know that positive communications are preferable to those that emphasize negative aspects (Wolpert et al. 2001, Lawson et al. 2008). Therefore, focusing on the positive, on resources, on shared perspectives lays a good foundation for building good relationships, which can contribute to the therapeutic alliance between operators and patients and treatment adherence.

2. TYPE I DIABETES: IMPACT OF THE DIAGNOSIS ON THE FAMILY

2.1. The Time of Communication of the Diagnosis

The diagnosis of Type 1 Diabetes Mellitus in a child puts the whole family in a complex situation.

Upon communication of the diagnosis, parents receive a lot of information and are called in a short time to acquire new skills related to their child's illness. Management of the disease requires new demands, which lead to the need to change the daily routine. Diabetes control requires planning different aspects of disease management, such as intervals between meals, blood glucose monitoring, administering insulin and inventory control, and finally physical activity. The complexity of management is compounded by the fear of ineffective blood glucose control, particularly in the form of hypoglycemia.

Along with the physiological risk that a parent assumes in raising a child, when he must accept to let him go, trusting that he has the resources to gradually become independent, other risks are added connected to the management of the disease and its form. Indeed, subjective interpretations shape the understanding of the disease outside the medical sphere: they mold the daily experience and also affect the relationship of others with the child and the procedures related to the management of the disease.

An element that can help to contain the concern is the accurate and adequate transmission of information. Since fantasies risk being more frightening than reality, particular care must be given to communication involving small children. In relation to cognitive development and the specific personal characteristics of patients, communication can use fairy tales, real objects or be articulated in more abstract and scientific terms. It is in any case important that instructions regarding how to measure blood glucose levels and to administer insulin are also given to patients; this can promote a closer-to-reality representation and a sense of responsibility, based on the characteristics of the patient.

A good adjustment is usually achieved after a year after diagnosis: if good glycemic control is reached, the family feels confident and the disease becomes easily integrated into family life. When, on the contrary, blood sugar is not well controlled, a sense of frustration and insecurity emerges (Cameron et al. 2005).

Three years after the diagnosis, the disease is described as a "natural element/component" of the family, although the possible fluctuation in blood sugar levels may still affect family life at various levels (Azar and Solomon 2001).

As time passes from the diagnosis, parents report that they have managed to adapt to the new routine and are confident in their Diabetes management skills, even if the feelings of loss, limitation of their freedom and fear for the future life of their child persist over time, even years after diagnosis. All interviewed parents consider it essential to have emotional support sources, both professional, such as health figures, and personal, such as friends, school staff and other parents in the same condition (Cameron et al. 2007).

Rankin and Lawton (2016), based on interviews with parents, have shown that, whether the diagnosis was recent or whether years had passed, the stories of parents of children with Type 1 Diabetes Mellitus were detailed and highly emotional. For some parents the experience of the diagnosis had been very distressing, as the disease in their child began with an episode of diabetic ketoacidosis. In others, instead, the sense of guilt had prevailed, as they felt responsible for the delay in the diagnosis, because they had underestimated the symptoms that their child presented. All parents were convinced they had "not done enough" and some reported that they had continued to brood, even for years, about the events that led to the diagnosis.

In the light of this, the importance is not only the screening of the parents of children with Type 1 Diabetes Mellitus for what concerns psychological distress (Cameron et al. 2007), but also continuous monitoring, due to the continuous dynamic equilibrium that the management of chronicity in the developmental age involves.

2.2. The Time of Chronicity

It is evident that the diagnosis of a single member actually has an impact on the whole family: in general, parents become anxious and also the siblings of the patients are at risk of developing behavioral disorders (Azar and Solomon, 2001).

In particular, parents find themselves having to psychologically adapt to a completely new condition (Drotar 1997) and are exposed to considerable levels of *stress,* since they must maintain their parental role and at the same time take care of their child, who has a chronic condition, with the need for continuous adherence and therapy (Streisand et al. 2001; Streisand et al. 2010).

The treatment of Diabetes Mellitus Type 1 requires not only continuous monitoring of blood glucose and insulin administration but also constant attention to physical activity and nutrition of the child (Drotar and Lewandoski 2007; Wysoki et al. 2009). The responsibility for these treatments, attributable to the parents, can alter family life, increasing the likelihood of maladjustment of the parents (Overstreet et al. 1995, De Beaufort and Barnard 2012) and, on the other hand, a well-balanced family affects the child's health (treatment adherence and blood glucose level control in the first place) (Cohen et al. 2004). In a systematic review, Whittemore et al. (2012) pointed out that the parents are primarily responsible for the daily management of the disease and this responsibility can contribute to aggravating stress and anxiety. Taking care of a child with Diabetes Mellitus is in fact an overwhelming experience, which requires constant attention (Sullivan et al. 2003) and raises concerns about episodes of non-glycemic control up to a real anxiety over the fear of death of the child (Mullins et al. 2004; Lowes et al. 2004).

The *stress* associated with managing the disease is due to several factors In particular, parents consider it difficult to maintain their child's blood sugar within certain limits: the *range* of values seems too close to them (Wennick 2006), they fear causing pain to their child whenever there is a need to monitor blood glucose and administer insulin (Marshall 2009), they feel the burden of "never being able to stop worrying" for their child, both about his current health and about possible long-term complications (Bowes 2009), they live with apprehension the moments of "Transition", such as the beginning of schooling and the transition from childhood to adolescence are lived with further apprehension (Ib.), finally they must organize new routines around the care of the loved one-patient, with risks of social isolation, which in adults can increase feelings of fear or frustration and feelings of guilt or helplessness, or both (Hatton 1995; Sullivan 2006).

Continuous *stress* and worry manifest themselves in the high prevalence of psychological distress reported by parents and in the increased risk of depression and anxiety: high levels of *stress* are indeed predictive of symptoms of anxiety and depression (Jaser et al. 2009;

Kovacs et al. 1990; Mitchell et al. 2009; Streisand et al. 2005; Streisand et al. 2008).

A study by Moreira et al. (2013) found higher levels of anxiety among parents of children with Type 1 Diabetes compared to parents of healthy children, understandably due to great responsibility in managing the disease and concern about the future, but, unlike other studies, no differences were found between the two groups regarding symptoms of depression. It should be noted that the study took into consideration a wider age range (8-18 years) compared to other studies and probably parents of children suffering from Diabetes for a long time could have developed effective strategies to meet the needs of the child, with a lower incidence of symptoms of depression. As a matter of fact, a comparative study has shown that parents of young children experience more anxiety than parents of older children or in any case with more years of illness (Stallwood 2005). A third useful aspect to explain the different responses is that depression is more closely associated with an experience of loss or a perception of self-depreciation, while anxiety is more linked to experience or perception of threat or danger (Beck et al. 1985). Once the grief for the loss of the healthy child has been elaborated, the parents preserve the concern for the unexpected linked to the disease, such as episodes of hypoglycemia. This portion of unpredictability combined with the complexity of the treatment regime contributes to the high levels of fear and anxiety in parents but does not equally affect symptoms of depression.

Parental discomfort affects family life in a different way depending on whether there are more symptoms of depression or more anxiety symptoms. Symptoms of depression are associated with inconsistency of discipline, less emotional warmth, less involvement and lower abilities to adapt and family cohesion, which translate into an increase in conflicts between family members; in addition, symptoms of depression are linked to less parental control of disease management (Eckshtain et al. 2010). The anxiety symptoms instead lead to a greater tendency to control and to maternal overprotectiveness and this implies a greater parental involvement in the management of Diabetes (Streisand et al. 2008; Cameron et al. 2007).

The mother has an important role within the family nucleus; since she is the parental figure who assumes the greatest responsibility for raising the child and also specifically for the disease, she is usually the primary caregiver in the treatment. Perhaps in light of such an investment, in various studies, it emerges that mothers of children with Type 1 Diabetes are at greater risk in developing anxiety and depressive symptoms and face greater stress (Horsch et al. 2007; Driscoll et al. 2010), which reflects on their parenting and therefore on the quality of life of the child and on his psychosocial adaptation (Jaser et al. 2009; Kovacs et al. 1990).

It is interesting to note that mothers report greater concern than fathers and above all a sense of loneliness (Horsch 2007). This sense of loneliness is also confirmed in another study (Driscoll et al. 2010), which shows that 6 months after the diagnosis they are disappointed by the lack of involvement of the father.

The understanding of the reason for this paternal "absence" is not so easy to explain. On the one hand, it shows how fathers need more time to adapt to the new situation of family life, on the other it would be the exclusivity of the mother-child relationship to generate in the fathers a feeling of exclusion and to support "avoiding" coping strategies (Azar and Solomon 2001).[*]

It would be interesting to investigate the extent to which avoidance strategies are able to contain anxiety or if, together with the experience of exclusion, they do not find expressions in other channels, for example in somatic symptoms or forms of addiction, such as the workaholic.

Even if the literature progressively moves towards a more systemic interpretation and not focused exclusively on the mother-child dyad, the primary social place, where daily activities related to treatment, but not only, are carried out, is often the mother-child dyad. So many studies have considered the maternal variable in its effects on health behaviors, even if

---

[*] A different feeling between fathers and mothers also emerges with respect to parents' satisfaction of the care received. The majority of parents are satisfied, both at the time of the diagnosis and afterwards (Azar and Solomon 2001), but mothers have reported less satisfaction than fathers, again due to the sense of loneliness they experience in caring for the child.

it is evident that the maternal role reflects the dynamics of the family and first of all the couple.

That being said, in literature we find that maternal difficulties in family relationships are predictive not only of poorer dietary adherence but also of potentially dangerous behaviors for the child's health, such as the refusal of food, nibbling, drinking instead of eating (Sullivan, Bolyai et al. 2003; Patton et al. 2006). Mothers with children suffering from chronic illness are characterized by a more destructive behavior (anger, quarrels with their partner) compared with mothers of healthy children (Borge et al. 2004).

Patton and colleagues (2006, 2009) have found that the use of parental imperatives and coercive modalities during meals is related to less glycemic control and less dietary adherence by the child (for example, not obeying to eat); instead if the mother, while planning the meal, involves the child and encourages commitment (for example suggests and makes questions), then this is associated to a smaller number of emotional and behavioral problems, an improved dietary regime and also an improved glycemic control.

The studies of Chisholm and Atkinson (2012) demonstrate how the most effective communication strategies in promoting engagement by the child are conveyed by the affective quality of parental communication, in particular, a positive maternal communication (more affectionate and full of praise) is correlated to favorable predictive outcomes, including better self-regulation and better collaboration with parental requests. Another essential element is the consistency between verbal and non-verbal messages

It is interesting to note that if the authors find confirmation that an incongruent maternal communication correlates with a poorer dietary adherence of the child, on the other hand, a relationship between positive maternal communication and optimal dietary adherence has not been demonstrated.

The explanation of this can be attributed to the fact that a child's commitment represents a continuum of behaviors, which concerns both individual, family and social context variables.

In particular, in pediatric literature there is substantial evidence that higher levels of family cohesion are associated with better results in terms of child management (Chisholm et al. 2007); the parents themselves experience less difficulty in the daily management of the disease and have less psychological distress (Edmonds et al. 2010), good cohesion is also correlated to better maternal control and determines fewer symptoms of depression (Wallander et al. 1989).

Even the parents of children with Type 1 Diabetes confirm the link between family cohesion and adaptation. Parents who perceive their family environment as supportive show better adaptation, less *stress* and fewer symptoms of depression and anxiety: it is precisely in the family environment where they receive emotional support because concerns about the disease can be shared among the various members. Parents also report a more positive assessment of the impact of the disease and their quality of life. However, it should be noted that parents with children with Type 1 Diabetes have lower levels of family cohesion, regardless of the age of the children, compared to parents of healthy children. (Drew, Berg and Wiebe 2010).

3. RELATIONS AND SOCIAL CONTEXT

A goal shared by carers, parents, and patients is to live an existence as normal as possible and this implies participation in social life, cultivating relationships, practicing sports, hobbies…

A significant element in the social context is the community's attitude towards the child with chronic illness and the social policies regarding the administration of drugs in the public environment: these are important factors that modulate relationships in everyday life.

Both in social contexts and in those of parents, ambivalent elements can be found. At the social level, today there are still forms of stigmatization linked for example to have to inject insulin in public, in the face of information campaigns that present the disease as an easily manageable condition.

As for parents, ambivalence emerges in talking about the child as a "normal" child, but on the other hand to claim the need for special care and protection. Despite the constant attempts to convince others that Diabetes is not a disease, they experience a sense of inadequacy and distrust, particularly when the child is alone in the company of friends and their parents ("It's hard for me to send my child at birthday parties, because the other parents are uncomfortable, I also don't know if they would know how to behave in an emergency"). This lack of trust is very evident in the relationship with the school environment: on the one hand, parents refuse to define Diabetes Mellitus as a disability, denying that their child is a child with special needs, on the other hand, they are aware that giving the child the label of "sick person" will give them more help and support. When they talk to teachers, they try to convince them that Diabetes is a normal aspect, which is an integral part of their child's life, and at the same time they emphasize the seriousness of the disease to guarantee the child the right protection in case of complications (Nurmi and Stieber-Roger 2012).

It is clear that parents cannot autonomously carry out the task of being informers and educators with respect to Diabetes for the school system. Meetings with health professionals, with particular attention to the psychological aspects of living with Diabetes Mellitus, can instead promote a positive approach to the management of the disease in the school environment attended by the child. This also has another advantage: it reduces the sense of loneliness of the parent, who can thus sense the availability and support of the school and health system.

The risk of closure or distrust of the environment is always possible, so all opportunities for collaboration and openness can be useful. In particular, we note the effectiveness of meetings and associations of families and diabetic patients. For parents and children, meetings with those who live similar experiences are precious; the experience of sharing, mutual recognition, the possibility of experiencing the help given and received are elements that support and promote resilience and trust (Nurmi and Stieber-Roger 2012).

4. COPING STRATEGIES AND DISEASE REPRESENTATIONS

Adaptation to a chronic disease cannot be completely explained by the severity of the disease, but in order to fully understand the processes and the variability of adaptation, it is necessary to consider the "modifiable risk factors" and the "factors of protection or resistance". (Wallander et al. 1992).

The "modifiable risk factors" include disease parameters, the efficacy of the treatment and psychosocial stressors. However, the "factors of protection or resistance" are the personal capacities that emerge in the face of illness, including the cognitive assessment of its impact on the family and the sense of change and mastery of the situation, perceived also thanks to aspects of family and social support.

Among the resistance, factors are included coping strategies, i.e., the set of cognitive and behavioral efforts implemented to control specific internal and/or external requests, which are evaluated as exceeding the person's resources. These intentional actions, both cognitive and behavioral that the person puts in place to control the negative impact of the stressful event, constitute a dynamic process, a series of reciprocal responses through which the environment and the individual influence each other.

There are two different types of *coping* (Karlsen et al. 2004):

- Problem-focused coping, which consists of trying to modify or resolve the situation that is threatening or damaging the individual
- Emotion-focused coping, which consists in the regulation of negative emotional reactions resulting from the stressful situation

Problem-focused coping strategies are generally used in situations perceived as controllable and are associated with more positive results, with greater psychological adaptation and greater self-regulation (Moss et al. 1996, Karlsen et al. 2004) and, as regards Diabetes Mellitus, also better glycemic control (Smari and Valtysdottir 1997).

Instead, Emotion-focused coping strategies are used in situations that the subject perceives as less susceptible to change (Carver et al. 1989).

In the case of Diabetes Mellitus, as in all diseases with high controllability (Zeinder and Endler 1996), there is confirmation in the literature that problem-focused coping strategies are more effective than emotion-focused strategies (Wennick 2006).

An interesting theme, connected to coping strategies and investigated in different studies, is the relationship with the representation of disease (Hagger and Orbell 2003, Kaptein et al. 2006).

It would appear that more positive representations of disease, such as beliefs about its controllability, are linked to Problem-focused coping, while negative visions, such as excessive attention to symptoms, complications and chronic illness, are associated with less useful coping strategies.

Disease representations are shaped by various factors, among which personality traits, education and personal experience of illness stand out.

As a matter of fact, research shows that coping processes are built on the interaction between personality traits and the surrounding environment (Parkers 1986).

Thus Lawson et al. (2010) studied how personality traits and interaction with the therapeutic environment can influence coping strategies in subjects with Diabetes Mellitus and how the perception of health messages is correlated with more or less adaptive strategies.

The data of the study confirm the results of previous research (Parkers 1986; Carver et al. 1989), in which it was evident how extroversion, emotional stability, open-mindedness and capacity for acceptance were correlated to Problem-focused coping strategies, or effective behaviors and "protective" towards their own health, such as planning and research of instrumental and emotional supports aimed at the desire to control the disease (Auerbach et al. 2002).

It is important to underline that these characteristics allow the subject to construct a mental representation of the most positive disease, where there is a better-perceived control; this directs the person towards the use of Problem-focused coping (Hagger and Orbell 2003).

The representation of disease therefore has a fundamental role as a mediator in coping strategies.

The authors noted that personality traits are predictive of how the perception of the disease varies, but the strongest predictor of disease representation is the way in which the disease is explained to the patient at the time of diagnosis.

The way in which the subject perceives the health message when the disease is communicated is of fundamental importance (Lawson et al. 2008). The perception of reassuring messages about the disease is related to its acceptance and to more active and Problem-oriented coping strategies. In fact, the subject perceives a greater possibility of glycemic control, both from the point of view of therapy and from the point of view of personal behavior. On the contrary, the perception of more threatening and less reassuring messages determines weaker emotional and behavioral responses, because the subject places attention on the severity of the disease and is less inclined to believe in the effectiveness of the treatment.

Contrary to expectations, however, it was seen that after two years the same subjects who had perceived the diagnosis as threatening, showed the same planning and research behaviors of emotional and instrumental supports as the patients who had perceived the news of illness as a reassuring message.

The explanation of this lies in the fact that Diabetes Mellitus, unlike other diseases, can be kept under control by the patient to a large extent by implementing lifestyle changes and self-care activities (diet, exercise, regular blood glucose control and self-administration of insulin).

But there are also different evidences. For example, in previous studies on Diabetes Mellitus Type 2, the perceptions of gravity were related to better self-management (Hampson et al. 1990, 1995). In fact, the perception of threatening messages seems to encourage people to seek support both instrumentally and emotionally.

It is possible that the data are only apparently divergent: it is important that the communication reflects the objective data and supports the patient's adherence. In the case of Diabetes, the severity reported by the doctor is often reflected in the patient's subjective perception and the doctor's communication mode is part of this reality. The communication according to the known indications of the acronym SPIKES (Buckman

2000) allow to reach the communication of the diagnosis in respect of the objective data, of the indications on the informed consent, of how much the patient already knows and how much he wants to know and in respect of the emotional state of the patient. Effective communication in the diagnostic phase is essential, although it should be foreseen that during the course of the illness it may be necessary to support the patient for the purposes of good personal control and the effectiveness of the treatment.

The periodic evaluation of the perception of illness and of coping strategies over time also helps the operators in planning education programs and/or interventions aimed at the use of coping strategies that are useful to this specific disease (Cameron et al. 2005).

5. MIDDLE CHILDHOOD

Middle childhood is the developmental period between early childhood and adolescence; on a psychological level, the child becomes increasingly independent, begins to renegotiate boundaries and relationships and above all begins to rely less on parents and to invest more on horizontal relationships with peers (Cincotta 2008).

The awareness of being carriers of a disease (whatever it may be) can place the preadolescent in a position of disadvantage compared to his/her companions: the risk is to deny the illness before his companions, considered as a weakness, a drawback and possible discrimination, to then pass on to deny even the treatments, which are the "obvious, public" part of the disease itself. It is not so much a question of safeguarding medical privacy, but rather of safeguarding one's own image, a point already in itself too easily vulnerable and purposefully sensitive in the psychology of the preadolescent.

The relationship between the young person and the caregiver is "transactional" (Sameroff et al. 2009), and this means that the characteristics and behaviors of the young and the caregiver influence and mutually shape each other (Sameroff and Mackenzie 2003). This has also been confirmed in the relationship between adolescents with Diabetes

Type 1 and their caregivers (Thompson and Gustfson 1996; Chaney et al. 1997; Hocking and Lochman 2005) and this relationship influences both adherence to the therapeutic regimen and blood glucose level control (Lewin et al. 2006), as well as family life (Anderson et al. 2002; Ellis et al. 2007).

The increasing autonomy of the preadolescent is also reflected in the progressive shift of responsibility for care from parents to the child (Anderson and Collier 1994). In this transition, it is important to maintain a good-quality parent-child relationship (Berg et al. 2011). In particular, a "critical" parent will deteriorate the quality of the relationship and compromise adherence ((Lewin et al. 2006, Sweenie et al. 2014), also in the transition from childhood to adolescence (Duke et al. 2008) Furthermore, this behavior of the parent leads to an increase in the frequency of symptoms of depression in the preadolescent stage and a lower efficacy in self-care (Armstrong et al. 2011).

There are three main parenting styles: authoritative, authoritarian and permissive. In the first, consistent but flexible limits are set and there is a high level of emotional warmth and emotional support; the authoritarian style is characterized by a high degree of control and the family environment is structured so as to give great importance to obeying the rules; finally in the permissive behavior there is a sensitivity to the emotional needs of the child, but in a poorly structured environment (Baumrind 1971). Literature indicates that authoritative parenting style is associated with positive results regarding child health, sports activities, healthy eating and lower risk of obesity and this can play a crucial role in the daily management of Type 1 Diabetes (Hubs-Tait et al. 2008; Wake et al. 2007; Rhee et al. 2006; Harris et al. 2001); even with regard to adolescents, authoritative parents contribute to a better glycemic control and also to an improved ability for self-care (Shorer et al. 2011). The warmth and affection of parents is also positively associated with better behavioral adherence even in younger children, aged between 4 and 10 years (Davis et al. 2001).

The parenting style during preadolescence was studied by Monaghan et al. (2012). The results of the study indicate that 97% of those tested used an authoritative parenting style, with reduced use of authoritarian style, and that only 3% used a permissive style. This style correlated positively with a better family life and better adherence of self-care behavior, but, contrary to other studies (Streisand 2005), parental stress was not significantly associated with less metabolic control or worse behavioral adherence, although a more authoritative parental behavior was associated with more positive responses to stress.

6. Middle Childhood: A Pilot Study

Middle childhood represents an age which is not much explored in the literature, compared to childhood and adolescence. Our research is aimed at this age group.

The aims of this pilot and observational study are to detect the levels of happiness and satisfaction of a sample of children with Type 1 Diabetes Mellitus and their parents and to qualitatively evaluate the way how their chronic experience is represented, taking account of the control and management of Type 1 Diabetes Mellitus.

6.1. Method

Subjected to the authorization of the provincial ethics committee (protocol No. 1880) and informed consent, patients and parents were contacted by telephone and then met in person at the pediatric Diabetes clinic, where they were able to compile the battery of tests separately.

6.1.1. Instruments

Values of glycated hemoglobin (previous-year-trend and current situation) recorded in medical records.

Self Care Inventory (La Greca A. 2004): the SCI is a 14-items self-report measure of behaviors associated with patients' perception of their adherence to Type 1 Diabetes self-care (La Greca, Swales, Klemp and

Madigan, 1988; La Greca and Bearman 2003). Respondents report on adherence behaviors using a 5-point scale. The items considered in the SCI are 5 and reflect the main components of the Type 1 Diabetes' regimen, including monitoring and recording glucose, administering and adjusting insulin, regulating meals and exercise and keeping appointments. Respondents report on their behaviors over a 2-weeks period. Scores are summed (a total score and a total for each subscale are gained) and divided by the total number of items in each scale (subtracting the number of items marked as "Not Applicable" from the dominator); values were then multiplied by 10 to provide a more conventional metric. Higher scores reflect more optimal adherence.

Subjective Happiness Scale (Lyubomirsky and Lepper 1999): The SHS is a self-report measure consisting of 4 items on a 7-step scale (from 1 = I am not a very happy person to 7 = I am a very happy person) who calculates subjective happiness. Among these, two items are aimed at evaluating the general perception of happiness and the other two assess the perception of their happiness in relation to peers. Three of the 4 items are formulated in a positive sense and one in the negative sense (whose score is calculated in the opposite direction). The total score is obtained by summing the individual items' scores and can go from 4 to 28. Higher scores represent a higher level of happiness. SHS has shown that it has sufficient internal consistency and test-retest reliability, a one-dimensional factorial structure and concurrent validity with various variables of emotionality and relationship (Lyubomirsky et al. 2011; Lyubomirksy and Lepper 1999). Therefore, it turns out to be a good tool for the assessment of subjective happiness. There are Italian translations and standardizations on an Italian sample (Iani et al. 2014).

Satisfaction With Life Scale (SWLS - Diener E. 1984): the SWLS is a 5-items self-report scale that measures the overall satisfaction of life. You are asked to respond to the items by compiling a 7-point Likert scale (from 1 = I strongly disagree, 7 = I completely agree). The total score is given by summing the items and can vary between 5 and 35. A high total score indicates a high level of overall satisfaction in life. It has been shown that SWLS is a psychometrically good tool to quickly measure life satisfaction, in fact, it has a strong internal reliability (r = 0.87) and moderate temporal stability (r = 0.82, two months of test-retest reliability) (Diener et al. 1984). There isn't an Italian version nor standardization on an Italian sample. Translation from English has been performed.

A short paper on the disease experience, according to Pennebaker works (1996, 2004). The patients and their parents were also asked to write respectively about their experience of the illness and about dealing with a diabetic child for ten minutes.

The SCI has been exclusively proposed to patients. Subjective Happiness Scale, Satisfaction With Life Scale and the short paper has been proposed to both parents and patients.

6.1.2. Sample

Recruitment criteria included patients with Type 1 Diabetes (at least 36 months), aged between 8 and 15 years, and the ability to read and to understand study materials. A consent form has been signed by each parent. We met 50 families. The patients, of which 58% males and 42% females, were between 8 and 15 years old (*M. = 12,36, Mdn = 13,* SD = 1,93).

Not all the subjects of the sample compiled all the proposed protocols.

Diabetology clinic is a reference point for the whole province and patients can reside tens of kilometers away. For this reason, we tried to carry out the research protocols during the days of already scheduled visits. However, this has affected the possibility for each subject to complete the test administration, so there are numerically different samples for the various tests. Also, not both parents were always present at the visits and the compiled-at-home protocols for the absent parents were rarely delivered. Subjects were not paid for their participation.

6.1.3. Statistical Analysis

Even if the data are numerical, they are actually ordinal, so non-parametric tests were applied; however, considering that the data are approximately normally distributed, the evaluations were also repeated with parametric tests. A series of correlations were made between the variables taken into consideration. The Mann-Whitney U test, t-test, and ANOVA test were performed. In the narratives, a quantitative analysis of the frequencies was conducted with the use of the NVIVO program as well as a qualitative analysis of the texts.

7. RESULTS

Regarding the evaluation of subjective happiness (SHS), the parents' scores are not inferior to those found in the Italian study by Iani et al. (2014) as well as patient data, although our sample is younger and the averages of the two samples do not show significant differences (SHS patient t (54) =. 051, $p = ns$; SHS mother t (237) = 1.25, $p = ns$; SHS father t (503) = 1.85, $p = ns$).

According to Pavot and Diener (2013) in relation to the assessments of the SWLS, both mothers and patients' groups fall within the upper limit of the score range (20 – 24). This result suggests "that they have areas of their lives that need improvement", while the fathers are placed in the next range (25-29). "Individuals who score in this range like their lives and feel that things are going well. Of course, their lives are not perfect, but they feel that things are mostly good." (see Table n°1)

By comparing the assessments of subjective happiness between patients and mothers, no statistically significant differences emerge (SHS t (76) =. 62, $p = ns$), as well as between patients and fathers (t (57) =. 92, $p = ns$). No statistically significant differences emerge even by comparing parents to one another - t (67) = .043, p = ns.

Also from the comparison of SWLS data, there are no differences between mothers and children: t (74) =. 53, $p = ns$; between mothers and fathers: t (64) = 1.66, $p = ns$; though not reaching it, we note that the averages of fathers and children tend to be significant: t (54) = 1.97, $p = .053$.

With respect to correlations, the statistically significant links between patient's SHS and SWLS are reported ($r = .482$, $p <.01$; $rho =. 386$, $p< .05$ two-tailed) as well as between mothers' SHS and SWLS ($r = .453$, $p <.01$;

rho =. 499, *p*‹ .01 two-tailed) and between mothers and children SHS (*r* = .496, *p* ‹.01; *rho* =. 535, *p*‹ .01 two-tailed).

Table 1. SHS and SWLS of patient, mother, and father

	SHSPt	SWLSPt	SHSM	SHSFr.	SWLSM	SWLSFr
N Valid	34	35	44	25	41	25
Average	4,9441	24,03	5,0966	5,2000	24,76	26,92
Median	5,0000	26,00	5,1250	5,0000	26,00	28,00
Mode	4,25	29	5,75	4,75	21	30
Std. Deviation	1,12248	6,331	1,02045	,99216	5,535	4,339

Considering the SCI data, the values have a range between 20 and 48.50, M = 37.80, *Mdn* = 39.25, SD = 6.16. Compared to data from Lewin et al. (2009), involving a sample aged 11-18 years, there are no significant differences (t (194) =. 71, $p = ns$).

From the correlation analysis between the SCI and the patient's SWLS, it emerges a statistically significant result: r = .583, p ‹.01; *rho* =. 605, p ‹.01 two-tailed. SCI is correlated to fathers' SWLS with non-parametric indicator (*rho* = 579, p ‹.05,), but not with Pearson's correlation (r = 547 p = *ns* two-tailed).

As regards to glycated hemoglobin (HbA1c), the values range from 6.6% (49 mmol/mol) to 11.50% (102 mmol/mol), M = 7.9% (63 mmol/mol), Mdn = 7.7% (61 mmol/mol), SD = 1.00. In our sample a good control of Diabetes, which we consider ≤ 7.5% (59 mmol/mol), is reached by 18 patients, a bad control (≥ 8%, 64 mmol/mol) by 17 patients and 15 patients are in the middle range.

HbA1c is correlated to patients' SWLS with non-parametric Pearson indicator (r = -.470, p ‹.01 two-tailed), but not with Spearman correlation (*rho* = -290, $p = ns$), while there is no correlation between SCI and HbA1c. (r = .26, $p = ns$; *rho* =.-29, $p = ns$ two-tailed).

No correlation was found for the following interactions: HbA1c and mothers' SWLS (r = -164, $p = ns$; *rho* =-.256, $p = ns$ two-tailed), HbA1c and fathers' SWLS (r = -205, $p = ns$; *rho* = -.162, $p = ns$ two-tailed), SCI and mothers' SWLS (r = .059, $p = ns$; *rho* =.005, p ns two-tailed), SCI and fathers' SWLS ($r = .467$, $p = ns$; $rho = .371$, $p = ns$ two-tailed), HbA1c and mothers' SHS ($r = .021$, $p = ns$; $rho = -.140$, $p = ns$ two-tailed), HbA1c and fathers' SHS ($r = .008$, $p = ns$; $rho = .007$, $p = ns$ two-tailed), HbA1c and patients' SHS ($r = -.085$, $p = ns$; $rho = -.166$, $p = ns$ two-tailed), SCI and mothers' SHS ($r = .200$, $p = ns$; $rho = -.208$, $p = ns$ two-tailed), SCI and patients' SHS ($r = 058$, $p = ns$; $rho = .048$, $p = ns$ two-tailed).

By evaluating the variables in samples differentiated by sex through the Mann-Whitney Texts U, only one significant difference in the SHS distribution of mothers ($U = .008$) was found. Instead, no significant differences were found in the mothers' SWLS ($U = .221$), fathers' SWLS ($U = .610$), patients' SWLS ($U = 837$), patients' SHS ($U = .901$), fathers' SHS ($U = .610$), patients' SCI ($U = .191$), HbA1c ($U = .879$).

The same hypotheses have been verified and confirmed with ANOVA analysis: mothers' SHS ($F(1,41) = 6,35$, $p = .016$. In particular, mothers of male children are happier ($M = 5.41$, $SD = 1.05$) than mothers of daughters (($M = 4.65$, $SD = .85$).

There is no difference between patients' SHS ($F (1.31) = .087$, $p = .770$, nor even in the evaluation of adherence - SCI ($F (1.29) = 2.34$, $p = .163$) - or in glycated hemoglobin), HbA1c ($F (1.47) =. 01$, $p = .90$).

Furthermore, there are no differences between the patients' SWLS ($F (1.32) = .42$, $p = .552$, fathers' SHS ($F (1.22) = .03$, $p = .862$), mothers' SWLS ($F (1.38)) = 2.02$, $p = .163$), fathers' SWLS ($F (1.22) = 65$, $p = .427$.

72 narratives were collected: 35 from patients, 36 from mothers, 18 from fathers.

The words of all the narratives of patients were counted with the NVivo 12 software.

Patients used a total of 926 terms and 2360 words; on average, each narrative was composed of 67 words. The vocabulary of the maternal narratives included 1011 terms, with a total of 2771 words; the average length of the narratives was 78 words. Fathers used a total lexicon of 739, a total of 1652 words and an average narrative length of 92 words. The words were then grouped into thematic areas.

The most common terms are related to Diabetes and illness (177); more specific terms of treatment, such as insulin, glycemia, and insulin pump occurred 52 times. Though using specific terms for treatment, the words "diagnosis" or "chronicity" are never used: it was therefore said "my child will be caught forever" instead of "my child has a chronic disease/pathology".

The reference to the debut was found in many stories and the terms referring to it occurred 43 times. Similarly, the terms comparing the current situation (now) appeared 42 times. Expressions that generally referred to time and change were 172. In general, expressions with positive connotations were 99 compared to the 60 negative ones. The terms indicating the presence of relationships were 68 and among these, families (18) and parents (17) were the most frequent ones.79 was the frequency of terms referring to coping, with verbs such as dealing with, reacting, accepting, living together. The superego theme (must, must) had a frequency of 27.

Causal links occurred 90 times; temporal adverbs 78; prepositions introducing different perspectives (though, despite, instead) were 28 and adverb adjectives indicating a modulation (hardly, almost, some, etc.) were used 37 times.

By evaluating the words used in the narratives of the patients and their two parents, we found that the most used term in the three groups was "not". The terms "Diabetes" or "disease" appeared as the second most used in patients, as the third in fathers and as the twelfth in mothers. The third most frequent term in patients' narratives was "why", which in mothers was in the eleventh position and in the eighth in fathers. Among the other most used terms, we found the term "better" in the ninth position in children, twenty-first in mothers thirteenth in fathers, the term "good" was the sixteenth in patients, eighteenth in mothers and seventeenth in fathers.

It is also interesting to note how the term "anxiety" appears in the narratives of mothers, but it is absent in those of fathers and children, while "trauma" is found in the narratives of fathers and it is absent in those of mothers and patients. The terms "fear" and "guilt", "I hope" are absent in the paternal narratives, but present in the other two groups.

In general, parents' narratives conveyed an intense emotional involvement, especially in the memory of the debut and a concern for the future and for the transition to adolescence. In some narratives, it was stressed that the illness had strengthened the bonds of the couple and/or family and presented images of the children as a "special" child: "more sensitive", "exceptional", "a superhero". In the patients' narratives there were less intense tones: more than a drama, they highlighted fatigue, limits, attention. In general, they were narratives in which the most operational dimension or the description of external events prevailed over emotional contact or introspection.

A constant concern of parents was linked to the possibility for the disease to be under control in order to avoid negative consequences. We, therefore, hypothesized that situations somehow alarming negatively affected the representation and the memories connected to the experience with a diabetic child, while the tranquility of the present could induce more serene narratives. By considering glycated hemoglobin values $\leq 7.5\%$ (59 mmol/mol and $\geq 8\%$, 64 mmol/mol), we divided the sample into two subgroups and evaluated the narratives of parents and patients. Fifteen parents' narratives belonged to the first subgroup and twenty-two to the second.

Some interesting differences emerged from the comparison. 68% of parents in the first subgroup wrote about the onset of the illness, while 40% of parents in the second subgroup talked about it. In the second subgroup, the communication of the diagnosis was narrated with sentences like "...the first moment of complete bewilderment and total despair", "the trauma fell on me", "an experience that was at the beginning traumatic and devastating"; in the first group, although these kind of expressions were also present, there were more metaphorical expressions and images, such as "as if they had given me a blow on the head", "a hurricane that overwhelmed me", "a bolt from the blue", "it seemed that the world had fallen on me", "like being hit by a running train". In this same group, the reference to the debut was often used to trace an evolutionary path, a trajectory, which, starting from a destabilizing situation, reached a situation of "serenity", of "tranquility". The recognition (not the negation) of difficulties or fatigue was present, but the tones were more moderate, balanced. In the second group, this evolutionary idea was scarcely present, rather there was either a sense of resignation, of helplessness, or a sort of rationalization, an appeal to the will such as "therefore it is useless to mull over it. You must always look ahead!", "... I try to carry it forward with dignity". Alongside this, there were some expressions of anger and guilt, which did not appear in the first group.

Compared to the narratives of child-children, nine were from patients with good control and ten with inadequate control of the disease. A salient element of the first group was the ability to narrate the situation with moderate tones and with the presence of positive and negative aspects: "I'm quite well", "but sometimes I don't feel like...", "(I like it both.) I like some aspects and don't like others. I like it because I have the dog, the phone and during the checks, I can call the mother. I don't because changing set and sensor, making blood sugar, making insulin are a pain". In the second group, there was a greater "polarization": on one hand, expressions like "by now... I live very well", "I am very well, I feel very self-confident", on the other, expressions of anger "but fuck I am normal, I do not have psychological or physical problems, it's just that my pancreas doesn't work as it should", or a sense of fatigue, of chronicity "Diabetes... busts my comps", "I find this disease very annoying...".

8. Discussion

Although the treatment of Diabetes is demanding and there are still risks related to possible hypoglycemia and hyperglycemia, it is interesting to note that, in the considered sample, the levels of subjective happiness and satisfaction of life did not differ from the population. Many are the visions of happiness and satisfaction; moreover, they are evaluated according to subjective criteria. It could be interesting to be able to verify if the experience of illness, while not modifying the quantitative evaluations, has promoted qualitative changes, perhaps accentuating the eudaimonial dimension on the hedonic one. One fact that could support this hypothesis is that indicators of good control and good management of the disease, such as the values of glycated hemoglobin and SCI, are not related to happiness and satisfaction, neither in fathers nor in mothers. In patients, on the other hand, these values are related to satisfaction; perhaps good control is also felt by patients as a personal success, which increases satisfaction, as well as being linked to a perception of better health, but which does not affect the perception of happiness in patients.

In the literature, it is reported that children and adolescents with Type 1 Diabetes are often non-adherent to physician recommendations (Anderson et al. 2002; Greening et al. 2007) and also in our sample we found a general difficulty of maintaining the glycated hemoglobin in an optimal range. Unlike the literature (Lewin et al. 2009, Quittner et al. 2002, 2008), the HbA1c values do not correlate with the patients' SCI assessment. This may be due to the fact that our sample has a lower age than those considered in the literature and that this may have affected the proper protocols compilation; furthermore, the criteria for the recruitment of our sample envisaged, unlike other studies, a diagnosis dated at least three years before; finally, it is not excluded that factors of psychological origin may have given rise to a bad control of the disease, even in the presence of an adherent regime (Andrade and Crésio 2019, Hagger 2018).

Concerning narratives, a rather good general picture emerges. According to the work of Pennebaker (1996, 1997), we can say that our sample can "narrate" its own experience. There is a good use of logical and causal links; there are negative terms, due to the fact that the experience of illness necessarily arouses sad, negative feelings, but there is also the ability to appreciate healthy and positive aspects of life, as evidenced both by the positive terms and by the use of adverbs which introduce different perspectives on events. Apart from the memory of the debut that still has many strong and dramatic accents in the parents, the general tone is calm, as evidenced not only by the qualitative reading but also by the number of modulating adjectives and adverbs. Even the high number of "not" used in the litotes contributes to dampening the tones. In the frequency of "not" expressions, one can also read, however, a way of contrasting other visions or readings: emblematic is the expression "I am not/ he's not ill". If we interpret it as a defense mechanism of denial, we can read all the difficulty of accepting this disease, which can allow an almost normal life, though still a chronic pathology. On the other hand, in these expressions, we can instead read the desire to claim a different identity from that of a sick person. A significant discriminant, which argues more in favor of denial or resilience, could be the more or less realistic representation of one's situation and the presence or absence of anger. This is reflected in the comparison of the narratives of patients whose control of glycated hemoglobin is good vs. negative. The use of mechanisms of negation (which are present as conscious forms of coping or as unconscious defense mechanisms) is accompanied in patients with tonal of manic, rather euphoric and somehow angry shades.

Even if the indicators in our possession are limited, we can think that even for parents a better situation (referred to children's hemoglobin), is accompanied by the capacity to represent a richer reality, both for the greater emotional contact, witnessed by the use of images, and for the temporal and evolutionary perspective. Undoubtedly, the experience of a diabetic child arouses emotions and affections in a parent, the discriminating factor is how these affects are lived. According to W. Bucci (1997), health, i.e., the integration of functions, the organization of behavior-oriented to a purpose and the establishment of a unitary sense of self, is linked to the ability to connect multiple representational formats of subsymbolic, non-verbal symbolic and verbal symbolic systems (referential process). The particular writing setting (with limited time and a task which was not repeatable over time) makes it difficult to access and describe one's emotions, so the ability to resort to images, according to the functioning of the non-verbal symbolic system, can report a good emotional-emotional contact.

Again, concerning emotions, the presence of words such as anxiety, fear, guilt, hope in the stories of mothers and not in fathers', can make one think of a greater difficulty in men to contact with their emotions, especially since the term trauma is instead present only in male stories, as if it indicated that the initial impact was equally strong. But apart from the limited data, a cultural factor certainly weighs in this, so the fact that fathers do not describe themselves as anxious or frightened does not mean that they are not.

CONCLUSION

The lives of patients with Type 1 Diabetes Mellitus and their parents is certainly demanding, but the disease does not affect either subjective happiness or satisfaction with life. The subjects of our sample, despite having different abilities to write (to elaborate?), concerning emotions and affections, show that they know how to narrate their own story, so that they can think and contain it in their mind and perhaps this is the reason why they live well, despite the difficulties.

ACKNOWLEDGMENTS

We thank the Department of Pediatrics - ASST Spedali Civili (director Prof. Alessandro Plebani) and in particular Dr. Elena Prandi for their collaboration. Thanks to Massimo Tognazzi for his contribution to the NVIVO analysis.

REFERENCES

Anderson, B. J., Auslander, W. F., Jung, K. C., Miller, J. P. and Santiago, J. V. (1990). Assessing family sharing of diabetes responsibilities. *Journal of Pediatric Psychology*, 15 (IV): 477-492.

Anderson, C. A. and Collier, J. A. (1994). Managing very poor adherence to medication in children and adolescents: an inpatient intervention. *Clinical Child Psychology and Psychiatry*, 4 (III): 393-402.

Anderson, B. J., Vangsness, l., Connel, A., Butler D., Goebel-Fabbri, A. and Laffel, L. M. (2002). Family conflict, adherence, and glycaemic control in youth with short duration type 1 diabetes. *Diabetic Medicine*, 19 (VIII): 635-642.

Andrade do Nascimento, C. J. and Crésio de Aragão, D. A. (2019). Influence of socioeconomic and psychological factors in glycaemic control in young children with type 1 diabetes mellitus. *Jornal de pediatria*, 95 (I): 48-53.

Armstrong, B., Mackey, E. R. and Streisand, R. (2011). Parenting behavior, child functioning and health behaviors in preadolescents with type 1 diabetes. *Journal of Pediatric Psychology*, 36 (IX): 1052-1061.

Auerbach, S. M., Clore, J. N., Kiesler, D. J., Orr, T., Pegg, P. O., Qick, B. G. and Wagner, C. (2002). Relation of diabetic patients health-related control and satisfaction with treatment. *Journal of Behavioural Medicine*, 25 (I): 17-31.

Azar, R. and Solomon, C. R. (2001). Coping strategies of parents facing child diabetes mellitus. *Journal of Pediatric Nursing*, 16 (VI): 418-428.

Baumrind, D. (1971). Current patterns of parental authority. *Developmental Psychology*, 4 (1p2), 1.

Beck, A. T., Emery, G. and Greenberg, R. L. (1985). *Anxiety Disorders and Phobias*. New York: Basic.

Berg, C. A., King, P. S., Butler, J. M., Pham, P., Palmer, D. and Wiebe, D. J. (2011). Parental involvement and adolescents' diabetes management: the mediating role of self-efficacy and externalizing and internalizing behavior. *Journal of Pediatrics Psychology*, 36 (III): 329-339.

Borge, A. I. H., Wefring, K. W., Lie, K. K. and Nordhagen, R. (2004). Chronic illness and aggressive behaviour: a population-based study of 4-years olds. *European Journal of Developmental Psychology*, 1 (I): 19-29.

Bowes, S., Lowes, L., Warner, J. and Gregory, J. W. (2009). Chronic sorrow in parents of children with type 1 diabetes. *Journal of Advanced Nursing*, 65 (V): 992-1000.

Bucci, W. (1997). *Psychoanalysis and Cognitive Science. A Multiple Code Theory*. New York, NY: Guilford Press.

Buckmann, R. (2000). SPIKES- A six –steps protocol for delivering bad news: applications to the patient with cancer. *The Oncologist*, 5 (IV): 302-311.

Cameron, L. D., Petrie, K. J., Ellis, C. J., Buick, D. and Weinman, J. A. (2005). Trait negative affectivity and responses to a health education intervention for myocardial infarction patients. *Psychology and Health*, 20 (I): 1-18.

Cameron, L. D., Young, M. J. and Wiebe, D. J. (2007). Maternal trait anxiety and diabetes control in adolescents with type 1 diabetes. *Journal of Pediatric Psychology*, 32 (VII): 733-744.

Carver, C. S., Scheier, M. F. and Weintraub, J. K. (1989). Assessing copies strategies: a theoretically based approach. *Journal of Personality and Social Psychology*, 56 (II): 267-283.

Chaney, J. M., Mullins, L. L., Frank, R. G., Peterson, L., Mace, L. D., Kashani J. H. and Goldstein D. L. (1997). Transactional patterns of child, mother, and father adjustment in insulin-dependent diabetes mellitus: a prospective study. *Journal of Pediatric Psychology*, 22 (II): 229-244.

Chisolm, V., Atkinson, L., Bayrami, L., Noyes, K., Payne, A. and Kelnar, C. (2012). An exploratory study of positive and incongruent communication in young children with type 1 diabetes and their mothers. *Child: Care, Health and Development*, 40 (I): 85-94.

Chisolm, V. Atkinson, L., Donaldson, C., Noyes, K., Payne, A. and Kelnar, C. (2007). Predictors of treatment adherence in young children with type 1 diabetes. *Journal of Advanced Nursing*, 57 (V): 482-493.

Cincotta, N. F. (2008). The journey of Middle Childhood- Who are "Latency-Age" Children? In *Developmental Theories Through the Life Cycle*, 2nd Ed., edited by Austrian SG: 79-132. New York, NY: Columbia University Press.

Cohen, D. M., Lumkley, M. and Naar-King, S. (2004). Child behavior problems and family functionings predictors of adherence and glycemic control in economically disadvantaged children with type 1 diabetes: A prospective study. *Journal of Pediatric Psychology*, 29 (III): 171-184.

Davis, C. L., Delamater, A., Shaw, K., La Greca, A. M., Eidson, M. S., Perez-Rodriguez, J. E. and Nemery, R. (2001). Parenting styles, regimen adherence, and glycemic control in 4- to 10- year-old children with diabetes. *Journal of Pediatric Psychology*, 26 (II): 123-129.

De Beaufort, C. and Barnard, K. (2012). Challenges to emotional well being. Depression, anxiety and parental fear of hypoglycemia. In *Psychosocial Aspects of Diabetes: Children, Adolescents and Their Families*, edited by Christie D. and Clarissa M.: 38-52. University of Louxembourg: CRC Press.

Diener, E. (1984). Subjective well-being. *Psychological Bulletin*, 95 (III): 542-575.

Diener, E., Emmons, R. A., Larsen, R. J. and Griffin, S. (1985). The satisfaction with life scale. *Journal of Personality Assessment*, 49 (I): 71–75.

Diener, E. and Seligman, M. E. P. (2002). Very happy people. *Psychological Science*, 13 (I): 81–84.

Drew, J. M. Berg, C. and Wiebe, D. J. (2010). The mediating role of extreme peer orientation in the relationships between adolescent-parent relationship and diabetes management. *Journal of Family Psychology*, 24 (III): 299-306.

Driscoll, K. A. (2010). Risk factors associated with depressive symptoms in caregivers of children with type 1 diabetes or cystic fibrosis. *Journal of Pediatric Psychology*, 35 (VIII): 814-822.

Drotar, D. (1997). Relating parent and family functioning to the psychological adjustment of children with chronic health conditions. What have we learned? *Journal of Pediatric Psychology*, 22 (II): 149-165.

Drotar, D. and Lewandoski, A. (2007). The relationship between parent-reported social support and adherence to medical treatment in families of adolescents with type 1 diabetes. *Journal of Pediatric Psychology*, 32 (IV): 427-436.

Duke, D. C., Geffken, G. R., Lewin, A. B., Williams, L. B., Storch, E. A. and Silverstein, J. H. (2008). Glycemic control in youth with type 1 diabetes: family predictors and mediator. *Journal of Pediatric Psychology*, 33 (VII): 719-727.

Edmonds-Myles, S., Tamborlane, W. V. and Grey, M. (2010). Perception of the impact of type 1 diabetes on low-income families. *Diabetes Educator*, 36 (II): 318-325.

Eckshtain, D., Ellis, D. A., Kolmodin, K. and Naar-King, S. (2010). The effects of parental depression and parenting practices on depressive symptoms and metabolic control in urban youth with insulin dependent diabetes. *Journal of Pediatric Psychology*, 35 (IV): 426-435.

Ellis, D. A., Podolski, C. L., Frey, M., Naar-re, S., Wang, B. and Moltz, K. (2007). The role of parental monitoring in adolescent health outcomes: impact on regimen adherence in youth with type 1 diabetes. *Journal of Pediatric Psychology*, 32 (VIII): 907-917.

Greening, L., Stoppelbein, L., Konishi, C., Jordan, S. S. and Moll, G. (2007). Child routines and youths' adherence to treatment for type 1 diabetes. *Journal of Pediatric Psychology*, 32 (IV): 437-447.

Hagger, M. S. and Orbell, S. (2003). A metanalytic review of the common-sense model of illness representations. *Psychology and Health*, 18 (II): 141-184.

Hagger, V., Hendrieckx, C., Cameron, F., Pouwer, F. and Skinner, T. C. (2018). Diabetes distress is more strongly associated with HbA1c than depressive symptoms in adolescents with type 1 diabetes: results from diabetes MILES Youth-Australia. *Pediatric Diabetes*, 19 (IV): 840-847.

Hampson, S. E., Glasgow, R. E. and Foster, L. S. (1995). Personal models of diabetes among older adults. Relationship to self-management and other variables. *Diabetes Educator*, 21 (IV): 300-307.

Hampson, S. E., Glasgow, R. E. and Toobert, D. J. (1990). Personal models of diabetes and their relations to self-care activities. *Health Psychology*, 9 (V): 632-646.

Harris M. A., Mertlich D. and Rothweiler J. (2001). Parenting children with diabetes. *Diabetes Spectrum*, 14 (IV): 182-184.

Hatton, D. L., Canam, C., Thorne, S. and Hughes, A. M. (1995). Parents' perception of the impact of caring for an infant or toddler with diabetes. *Journal of Advanced Nursing*, 22 (III): 569-577.

Hocking, M. C. and Lochman, J. E. (2005). Applying the transactional stress and coping model to sickle cell disorders and insulin-dependent diabetes mellitus: identifying psychosocial variables related to adjustment and intervention. *Clinical Child and Family Psychology Review*, 8 (III): 221-246.

Horsch, A., McManus, F., Kennedy, P. and Edge, J. (2007). Anxiety, depressive and post traumatic symptoms in mothers of children with type 1 diabetes. *Journal of Traumatic Stress*, 20 (V): 881-891.

Hubbs-Tait, L., Kennedy, T. S., Page, M. C., Topham, G. L. and Harrist, A. W. (2008). Parental feeding practices predict authoritative, authoritarian, and permissive parenting style. *Journal of American Diabetes Association*, 108 (VII): 1154-1161.

Iani, L., Lauriola, M., Layous, K. and Sirigatti, S. (2014). Happiness in Italy: translation, factorial structure and norming of the subjective happiness scale in a large community sample. *Soc. Indic. Res.*, 118 (III): 953-967.

Jaser, S. S., Whittemore, R., Ambrosino, J. B., Lindemann, E. and Grey, M. (2009). Coping and psychosocial adjustment in mothers of young children with type 1 diabetes. *Child Health Care*, 38 (II): 91-106.

Kaptein, A. A., Helder, D. I., Scharloo, M., Van Kempen, G. M. J., Weinman, J., Van Houwelingen, H. J. C. and Raymund, A. C. R. (2006). Illness perceptions and coping explain well-being in patients with Huntington's disease. *Psychology and Health*, 21 (IV): 431-446.

Karlsen, B., Idsoe, T., Hanestad, B. R., Murberg, T. and Bru, E. (2004). Perception of support, diabetes-related coping and psychological well-being in adults with type 1 and type 2 diabetes psychology. *Health and Medicine*, 9 (I): 53-70.

Kovacs, M., Iyengar, S., Goldston, D., Obrosky, D. S., Stewart, J. and Marsh. J. (1990). Psychological functioning among mothers of children with insulin-dependent diabetes mellitus: a longitudinal study. *Journal Consulting Clinical Psychology*, 58 (II): 189-195.

La Greca, A. M (2004). *Manual for Self-Care Inventory*. Miami- Fl: University of Miami- local.psy.miami.edu.

La Greca, A. M., Bearman, K. J. and Roberts, M. C. (2033). Adherence to pediatric treatment regimens. In *Handbook of Pediatric Psychology* (*3rd ed.*): 119-140. New York, NY: Guilford Press.

La Greca, A. M., Follannsbee, D. S. and Skyler, J. S. (1995). Adolescents with diabetes: gender differences in psychosocial functioning and glycemic control. *Children's Health Care*, 24 (I): 61-78.

La Greca, A. M., Swales, T., Klemp, S. and Madigan, S. (1988). Self care behaviors among adolescents with diabetes. *Ninth Annual Sessions of the Society of Behavioral Medicine (Abstract)* A42.

Lawson, V. L., Bundy, C., Belcher, J. and Harvey, J. N. (2010). Mediation by illness perceptions of the effect of personality and health threat communication on coping with the diagnosis of diabetes. *British Journal of Health Psychology*, 15 (III): 623-642.

Lawson, V. L., Bundy, C. and Harvey, J. N. (2008). The development of personal models of diabetes in the first two years from diagnosis. A prospective longitudinal study. *Diabetic Medicine*, 25 (IV): 482-490.

Lewin, A. B., Heidgerken, A. D., Geffken, G. R., Williams, L. B., Storch, E. A., Gelfand, K. M. and Silverstein, J. H. (2006). The relation between family factors and glycemic control: the role of diabetes adherence. *Journal of Pediatric Psychology*, 31 (II): 174-183.

Lewin, A. B., LaGreca, A. M., Gary, R., Geffken, L. B., Williams, D. C., Duke, E. A., Storch, J. H. and Silverstein, J. H. (2009). Validity and reliability of an adolescent and parent rating scale of type 1 diabetes adherence behaviors: the self-care inventory (SCI). *Journal of Pediatric Psychology*, 34 (IX): 999–1007.

Lowes, L., Lyne, P. and Gregory, J. W. (2004). Childhood diabetes: parents experience of home management and the first year following diagnosis. *Diabetic Medicine*, 21 (VI): 531-538.

Lyubomirsky S. and Lepper H. S. (1999). A measure of subjective happiness: preliminary reliability and construct validation. *Social Indicators Research*, 46 (II): 137-155.

Mackey, E. R., Hilliard, M. E., Berger, S. S., Streisand, R., Chen, R. and Holmes, C. (2011). Individual and family strengths. An examination of the relation disease management and glycemic control in youth with type 1 diabetes. *Families, Systems and Health*, 29 (IV): 314-326.

Manfredi, P. (2017). Can you live happily with a chronic illness? *Gazzetta Medica Italiana- Archivio per le Scienze mediche, January-February*, 176 (I-II): 57-66.

Manfredi, P. (2018). Aderenza e alleanza: osservazioni psicoanalitiche al servizio della medicina. *Recenti Progressi in Medicina* 2018, Apr, 109 (IV): 226-235. [Adherence and alliance: psychoanalytic observations at the service of medicine. *Recent Progress in Medicine* 2018, apr, 109 (IV): 226-235].

Marshall, M., Carter, B., Rose, K. and Brotherton, A. (2009). Living with type 1 diabetes: perception of children and their parents. *Journal of Clinic Nursing*, 18 (XII): 1703-1710.

Monaghan, M., Horn, I. B., Alvarez, V., Cogen, F. R. and Streisand, R. (2012). Authoritative parenting, parenting stress, and self-care in preadolescents with type 1 diabetes. *Journal of Clinical Psychology in Medical Settings*, 19 (III): 266-261.

Moreira, H., Frontini, R., Bullinger, M. and Canavarro, M. C. (2013). Caring for a child with type 1 diabetes: link between family cohesion, perceived impact, and parental adjustment. *Journal of Family Psychology*, 27 (V): 731-742.

Moss-Morris, R., Petrie, K. J. and Weinman, J. (1996). Functioning in chronic fatigue syndrome: do illness perceptions play a regulatory role? *British Journal of Health Psychology*, 1 (I): 15-25.

Mullins, L. L., Fuemmeler, B. F, Hoff, A., Chaney, J. M., Van Pelt, J. and Ewing C. A. (2004). The relationship of parental overprotection and perceived child vulnerability to depressive symptomatology in children with type 1 diabetes mellitus: the moderating influence of parenting stress. *Child Health Care*, 33 (I): 21-34.

Nurmi, M. A. and Stieber-Roger, K. (2012). Parenting children living with type 1 diabetes. A qualitative study. *The Diabetes Educator*, 38 (IV): 530-536.

Overstreet, S., Goins, J., Chen, R., Holms, C. S., Greer, T., Dunlap, W. P. and Frentz, J. (1995). Family environment and the interrelation of family structure, child behavior, and metabolic control for children with diabetes. *Journal of Pediatric Psychology*, 20 (IV): 435-477.

Parkers, K. R. (1986). Coping in stressful episodes: the role of individual differences, environmental factors, and situational characteristics. *Journal of Personality and Social Psychology*, 51 (VI): 1277-1292.

Patton, S. R., Dolan, L. M. and Powers, S. W. (2006). Mealtime interactions relate to dietary adherence and glycemic control in young children with type 1 diabetes. *Diabetes Care*, 29 (V): 1002-1006.

Pavot, W. and Diener, E. (2013). *The satisfaction with life scale (SWL). Measurement instrument database for the social science.* Retrieved from http: //www.midss.org/sites/default/files/understanding_swls_scores.pdf

Pennebaker, J. W. (2004). *Scrivi Cosa Ti Dice il Cuore. Autoriflessione e Crescita Personale attraverso la Scrittura di Sé.* Trento: Edizioni Erickson. [*Write what your heart tells you. Self-reflection and Personal Growth through the Writing of Self.* Trento: Erickson Editions].

Pennebaker, J. W. and Francis, M. (1996). Cognitive, emotional, and language processes in disclosure. *Cognition and Emotion*, 10 (VI): 601-626.

Quittner, A. L., Espelage, D. L., Levers-Landis, C. and Drotar, D. (2002). Measuring adherence to medical treatment in childhood chronic illness: considering multiple methods and sources of information. *Journal of Clinical Psychology in Medical Settings*, 7 (I): 41–54.

Quittner, A. L., Modi, A.C., Lemanek, K. L., Levers-Landis, C. and Rapoff, M. A. (2008). Evidence-based assessment of adherence to medical treatments in pediatric psychology. *Journal of Pediatric Psychology*, 33 (IX): 916–936.

Rankin, D. and Lawton, J. (2016). Parental response to a diagnosis of type 1 diabetes. *Journal of Family Health*, 26 (III): 32-35.

Rhee, K. E., Lumen, J. C., Appugliese, D. P., Kaciroti, N. and Bradley, R. H. (2006). Parenting styles and overweight status in first grade. *Pediatrics*, 117 (VI): 2047-2054.

Sameroff, A. (2009). The transactional model. In *Transactional Model of Development: How Children and Context Shape Each Other*, edited by

Sameroff A.: 3-21. Washington, DC, Us: American Psychological Association.

Sameroff, A. J. and Mackenzie, M. J. (2003). Research strategies for capturing transactional models of development: the limits of the possible. *Development and Psychopathology*, 15 (III): 613-640.

Shorer, M., David, R., Shoenberg-Taz, M., Levavi-Lavi, I., Phillip, M. and Meyerovitch, J. (2011). Role of parenting style in achieving metabolic control in adolescents with type 1 diabetes. *Diabetes Care*, 34 (VIII): 1735-1737.

Smari, J. and Valtysdottir, H. (1997). Dispositional coping, psychological distress and disease-control in diabetes. *Personality and Individual Differences*, 22 (II): 151-156.

Stallwood, L. (2005). Influence of caregiver stress and coping on glycemic control of young children with diabetes. *Journal of Pediatric Health Care*, 19 (V): 293-300.

Streisand, R., Braniecki, S., Tercyak, K. P. and Kazak, A. E. (2001). Childhood illness-related parenting stress: the pediatric inventory for parents. *Journal of Pediatric Psychology*, 26 (III): 155-162.

Streisand, R., Mackey, E., Elliot, B. M., Mednick, L., Slaughter, I. M., Turek, J. and Austin, A. (2008). Parental anxiety and depression associated with caring for a child newly diagnosed with type 1 diabetes: opportunities for education and counseling. *Patient Education and Counselings*, 73 (II): 333-338.

Streisand, R., Mackey, E. and Herge, W. (2010). Associations of parent coping, stress, and well-being in mothers of children with diabetes: examination of data from a national sample. *Maternal and Child Health Journal*, 14 (IV): 612-617.

Streisand, R., Swift, E., Wickmark, T., Chen, R. and Holmes, C. S. (2005). Pediatric parenting stress among parents of children with type 1 diabetes: the role of self-efficacy, responsibility, and fear. *Journal of Pediatric Psychology*, 30 (VI): 513-521.

Sullivan-Bolyai, S., Deatrick, J., Gruppuso, P., Tamborlane, W. and Grey, M. (2003). Constant vigilance: mothers' work parenting young children with type 1 diabetes. *Journal of Pediatric Nursery*, 18 (I): 21-29.

Sullivan-Bolyai, S., Rosenberg, r. and Bayard, M. (2006). Fathers' relations on parenting young children with type 1 diabetes. *American Journal of Maternal and Child Nursing*, 31 (I): 24-31.

Sweenie, R., Mackey, E. R. and Streisand, R. (2014). Parent-child relationships in type 1 diabetes: associations among child behavior, parenting behavior, and pediatric parenting stress. *Families, Systems and Health*, 32 (I): 31-42.

Thompson, R. J. Jr. and Gustafson, K. E. (1996). *Adaptation to Childhood Chronic Illness*. Washington, D.C. US: American Psychological Association.

Wake, M., Nicholson, J. M., Hardy, P. and Smith, K. (2007). Preschooler obesity and parenting styles of mothers and fathers australian national population study. *Pediatrics*, 120 (VI): e1520-e1527.

Wallander, J. L. and Varni, J. W. (1998). Effects of pediatric chronic physical disorders on child and family adjustment. *Journal of Child Psychology and Psychiatry*, 39 (I): 29-46.

Wallander, J. L. and Varni, J. W. (1992). Adjustment in children with chronic physical disorders: programmatic research on disability-stress-coping model. In *Stress and Coping in Child Health*, edited by LaGreca A. M., Siegal J. L., Wallander J. L. and Walker C. E.: 279-298. New York, NY: Guilford Press.

Wennick, A. and Hallstrom, I. (2006). Swedish families' lived experience when a child is first diagnosed as having insulin-dependent diabetes mellitus: an ongoing learning process. *Journal of Family Nursing*, 12 (IV): 368-389.

Whittemore, R., Jaser, S., Chao, A., Myoungock, J. and Grey, M. (2012). Psychological experience of parents of children with type 1 diabetes. A systematic mixed-studies review. *Diabetes education*, 38 (IV): 562-577.

Wiebe, D. J. Chow, C. M., Palmer, D. L., Butner, J., Osborn, P. and Berg, C. A. (2014). developmental processes associated with longitudinal declines in parental responsibility and adherence to type 1 diabetes management across adolescence. *Journal of Pediatric Psychology*, 39 (V): 532-541.

Wolpert, H. A. and Anderson, B. J. (2001). Management of diabetes: are doctors framing the benefits from the wrong perspective? *British Medical Journal*, 323 (VIICCCXIX): 994-996.

Wysoki, T., Buckloh, L. and Greco, P. (2009). The Psychological Context of Diabetes Mellitus in Youth. In *Handbook of Pediatric Psychology* (4th ed.) edited by Roberts M.C. and Steele R.G.: 287-302. New York, NY: Guilford Press.

Wysocki, T., Taylor, A., Hough, B. S., Linscheid, T. R., Yeates, K. O. and Naglieri, J. A. (1996). Deviation from developmentally appropriate self-care autonomy. Association with diabetes outcomes. *Diabetes Care*, 19 (II): 119-125.

Zehnder, M. and Eindler, N. S. (1996). *Handbook of Coping Theory, Research and applications.* New York: John Wiley.

In: Coping with Chronic Illness   ISBN: 978-1-53616-775-7
Editor: Meghan Mendoza   © 2020 Nova Science Publishers, Inc.

Chapter 2

INTERNALIZING/EXTERNALIZING SYMPTOMS, COPING PROFILES AND ADJUSTMENTS TO RECURRENT PAIN IN PEDIATRIC CANCER PATIENTS: A MIX-METHOD APPROACH

Alessandro Failo[1,], PhD, Francesca Nichelli[2], MS,
Momcilo Jankovic[2], MD and Paola Venuti[1], PhD*
[1]Department of Psychology and Cognitive Sciences,
University of Trento, Rovereto, Italy
[2] Hemato-oncology Outpatient Clinic of the Pediatric Clinic,
MBBM Foundation, San Gerardo Hospital, Monza, Italy

ABSTRACT

Pain management is a growing concern in pediatric cancer patients as pain can originate from multiple sources and negatively influence long-term children well-being. To gain a better understanding of the pain adjustment processes occurring in these young patients, here we have analyzed a cohort of 30 children and early adolescents with acute

* Corresponding Author's E-mail: a.failo@unitn.it.

leukemia or lymphoma facing cancer-related pain, focusing on the various coping strategies at different stages of therapy. Specifically, through a mix-method approach integrating quantitative and qualitative data, we have characterized a number of coping profiles, internalizing/externalizing symptoms and adjustment difficulties specific for children experiencing cancer-related pain. Altogether, these findings provide a framework with which to predict children at risk of developing maladjustments, in dare need of parent-focused psychosocial interventions.

Keywords: treatment-related pain, cancer, coping skills, internalizing/ externalizing symptoms, emotional adjustment, children, pediatrics, projective drawings

INTRODUCTION

Currently, the risk of developing cancer in childhood is around 1 in 500 worldwide, with acute lymphoblastic leukemia (ALL) being the most common hematologic malignancy [1]. Specifically, ALL accounts for 70% of all leukemia cases, the vast majority of which are diagnosed at a young age and require lengthy treatments, causing severe family burden [1, 2].

Over the past few decades, scientific advancements have increased the overall 5-year survival rate of all cancers to over 80% [1]. However, cancer therapies can be extremely harmful to young patients because they are administered at a time of significant growth and development of the body, which lays the foundations for subsequent overall adjustment and functioning.

Treatment options for childhood cancer generally include chemotherapy, radiation therapy, surgical resection, antibody infusion, and/or bone marrow/stem cell transplantation [3], even though their single or combined use strictly depends on which type of cancer is being treated. What does not seem to change among the different types of cancer is the length of the treatment they require, which can take up months or years of a child's life [4].

Children and adolescents with cancer are thus confronted with many challenges as their lives and routines are frequently being disrupted by hospital visits and repeated invasive and painful treatment procedures. As a result, pediatric cancer patients experience a profound disconnect with same-age peers and have poor school attendance, with a detrimental effect on their typical learning path and socialization experiences [5]. These different aspects during the whole treatment process jeopardize the well-being of a child by disrupting its emotional and behavioral adjustment [6-9].

A child's adjustment to a series of stress periods—from diagnosis to treatment and recovery—is characterized by specific internalizing and externalizing behaviors [6]. Thus, it is extremely important to identify behavioral maladjustments at early phases of active treatment due to their negative influence on long-term adaptation [10].

Despite some controversial findings, there is consensus that pediatric cancer patients are generally characterized by reduced autonomy, poor psychological status, reduced self-esteem and depression, especially during the first 3 to 6 months after cancer diagnosis. Intriguingly, these dimensions seem to improve after 6 months from diagnosis, and more so after completion of the first year of treatment [11].

The variability of findings in children coping with cancer-related pain highlights the importance of identifying those risks and protective factors determining positive and negative emotional adjustments, respectively [6]. Despite the scarcity of studies on the longitudinal trajectories of adaptation to cancer in pediatric patients, it is becoming increasingly evident how crucial this information can be to identify children with maladaptive adjustment trajectories in dare need of psychosocial interventions [10].

As it hinders adjustment, pain is becoming a growing concern in childhood cancer management [12]. Indeed, the vast majority of pediatric cancer patients will experience pain at some point in time during their cancer trajectory [13, 14]. In this regard, a survey of a heterogeneous population of children with cancer aged 10-18 years has shown pain to be the most prevalent symptom among inpatients [15].

In cancer patients, pain can originate from multiple sources such as the malignancy itself (e.g., pain associated with bone metastases) and all ensuing diagnostic and treatment procedures (e.g., venous punctures, spinal punctures, bone marrow biopsies and chemotherapy). However, a number of studies concur that children with cancer generally experience more pain from the diagnostic and treatment procedures rather than from the disease itself [16-18].

To make matters worse, pain can be exacerbated by fear, anxiety and uncertainty, all leading to enhanced emotional distress [19]. Furthermore, recurrent or chronic pain can increase the vulnerability of children to psychological consequences of unrelieved pain, such as post-traumatic stress disorder, anxiety and depression, thereby hampering their pain-coping efforts [20]. Thus, in light of the aforementioned, the relationship between pain and negative emotions should be regarded as reciprocal rather than unidirectional, that is to say that pain and psychological distress exert an equal adverse influence on one another [21].

Children experience pain in different ways according to the following variables: previous pain experiences, beliefs, sociocultural context, temperament, coping skills, emotional functioning and situation at the time. The direct expression of pain or a partial denial of it is often a consequence of these factors [22]. Thus, the assessment of feelings or emotions, which is essentially a subjective attribution, is extremely important as it pertains to the causes and consequences of relevant phenomena such as coping, externalizing/internalizing symptoms, social activity and well-being [23]. In this regard, it is widely accepted that children are able to accurately recall painful experiences, understand the logical nature of pain causality, and associate pain with particular feelings, such as anger, fear, anxiety and embarrassment [12]. A child's view on the function and consequences of pain may therefore influence the development of specific coping processes and beliefs. While a child's coping strategy is an active process aimed to achieve personal control over the stressful aspects of the environment and emotional status [24], a child's own belief, especially when the pain is perceived as a threat, can exacerbate and intensify the cancer-related pain experience. Additionally, as the impact of pain on the child's functioning increases, its perceived uncontrollability further amplifies the child's pain perception [21]. For instance, a child perceiving a certain treatment as discomforting and unnecessary, or rather considering it as a punishment, may tend to blow the situation out of proportion and experience more pain due to augmented stress and fear. On the other hand, a child who understands the usefulness of a procedure may adjust better to pain by focusing on the benefits of the treatments instead of its adverse effects [12].

Another important determinant of adjustment to pain in pediatric cancer patients is the parent-child interaction. From a symbolic interactionist theoretical perspective, this active interaction can indeed help both parents and children better define the situation and improve their coping behaviors [16]. Conversely, cancer-related pain is often positively associated with parental distress responses [25]. This can probably be ascribed to the bidirectional nature of the parent-child relationship given that persistent parental distress can negatively impact the child's well-being as well as the overall parents' adjustment to the treatment process [25, 26].

However, despite the important role played by parent-child interactions in cancer coping schemes, the vast majority of studies in childhood cancer have mainly investigated family relations rather than focusing on those between parents and children [27].

In light of the multiple dimensions involving the phenomenon of pain in childhood cancer, this study aims to explore the pain coping strategies of children and adolescents suffering from acute leukemia or lymphoma.

The first goal of this study was to compare the emotional characteristics of children with cancer to those of a control group of healthy children by means of the Draw-a-Person (DAP) test, using all 30 Koppitz emotional indicators (EIs) [28, 29]. We also aimed to determine the sense of family as an internalized system of relations through the Draw-A-Family (DAF) test, as described previously [30].

We hypothesized that the different child's self-representations and the coding categories for family figure drawings could provide important information regarding a child's self-perception and perception of the surrounding environment as a network of interconnected relationships. We also hypothesized that the number and the type of EIs would be different between the two groups, consistent with previous studies in patients with other disorders [31-33].

The second aim of this survey was to characterize the clinical profiles of pediatric cancer patients coping with pain during or following anticancer therapy using a mix-method approach so as to determine which factors put children more at risk for chronic pain. Our central hypothesis was that coping factors and emotional well-being would be associated with the children's perception of support provided by their parents during and after treatment. Given the scarce information available, we also assumed that the various phases of chemotherapy treatment would be associated with different coping skills and emotional traits.

METHODS

Setting, Participants and Procedures

This study was conducted at the Hemato-Oncology Outpatient Clinic and the Department of Pediatrics at University of Milan-Bicocca, Monza, Italy. Thirty children aged 7-14 years were enrolled in this observational study of a single cohort of pediatric patients suffering from one of the following hematological malignancies: acute lymphocytic leukemia (ALL), acute myeloid leukemia (AML), Hodgkin's lymphoma or non-Hodgkin's lymphoma.

Participants were excluded from the study if they were not Italian mother tongue or had been diagnosed with specific developmental delays. Following enrollment, no families withdrew from the study, and no adverse events were reported.

Participants in the control group—only for the projective test section—were randomly recruited from schools in the city of Rovereto. The inclusion criteria for the control group were as follows: healthy children with no medical complications whose age would match the age range of the children enrolled in the clinical group.

The procedure was fully explained to the children and their parents. Informed consent was obtained from all participants in accordance with the local institutional review board (IRB) approved protocol. All participants had access to psychosocial care according to hospital standards and guidelines.

Research Instrument and Measures

In order to understand how recurrent pain affected children with hematological malignancies from a psychosocial standpoint, we assumed that noninvasive and discrete testing may be the best suited approach, particularly when attempting to identify emotional distress in children and young adolescents.

Demographics

All demographic and medical information was gathered from psychosocial and medical records and included the following data: age, gender, time since diagnosis, type of hematological cancer, type and phase of treatment, relapse occurrence, hospital admission and ongoing medical intervention. Sociodemographic characteristics of the child's mother and father were the following: age, education level, employment status, occupation, other concomitant problem and presence of siblings. The socioeconomic status (SES) of the parents was calculated with the Four-Factor Index of Social Status [34-35] (Table 1).

Pain Intensity

Children used the numerical rating scale (NRS-11) to rate their current pain and average of all pain episodes during hospitalization. Children rated their pain using two scales with the following prompts: *"How much pain do you have now?"* and *"How much pain have you had on average during hospitalization?"* This scale is the most frequently used for children older than 7 years [36].

Questionnaire Related to Social Variables and Dyadic Interactions during Episodes of Pain

This questionnaire specifically developed by our research group—adapted from a version published by Mathews [37]—was administered to 2 psychologists assisting the families during the illness course. The psychologists met to discuss the interactions and eventual coding discrepancies. The measure included five specific subscales: 1) School attendance on a 3-point scale, scored from 1 "yes, with regularity," 2 "not always," 3 "no, just hospital school." 2) Constancy of support from friends and classmates during hospitalization, scored on a 3-point scale. 3) Explanations provided by health professionals during the therapies or painful procedures (scored from 1 to 3). 4) Observed parental acceptance of the child's emotions during painful episodes. The psychologists rated the parent's reactions—usually those of the mothers—to their children's emotional expressions, scored on a 5-point scale. Higher scores indicated reactions to the child's emotional expressions characterized by openness, acceptance, emotional availability and validation of the child's emotions and point of view. Conversely, lower scores indicated non-accepting reactions to the child's emotional expressions characterized by dismissing or distressed reactions, emotional unavailability and lack of validation of the child's emotions and point of view. 5) Observed quality of parent's advice provided to the child when he/she had to face pain, scored on a 5-point scale. Higher scores indicated parent advice characterized by encouragement for active problem solving to cope with pain, showing confidence in the child's ability to effectively dealing with the situation. Conversely, lower scores were indicative of lack of encouragement and confidence in the child's ability to handle the situation. Finally, at the end of the questionnaire we left a blank space for additional comments.

Observation during Protocol-Interview

During the entire interview process, the researchers took notes describing the type of behavioral attitude of each child while receiving instructions, answering the questionnaire and drawing (e.g., refusal, excessive speed, anxiety, concerns etc.) (adapted from Roberti [38]). The children's behaviors were listed in four categories: 1) Collaborative/ exploratory: the child showed curiosity and openness toward the tests). 2) Collaborative/non exploratory: the child worked quietly but lacked self-perception, providing evasive answers and developing a rigid and controlled behavior. 3) Resistant: the child showed doubts and misgivings towards the test, making statements such as *"Why do I need this test?"* or *"I do not believe in this test."* 4) Refusing: the child refused to participate and exhibited verbal assault or behaved in a passive-aggressive way.

Pain-Coping Skills

Pain-coping skills were assessed by the Waldron/Varni Pediatric Pain Coping Inventory (PPCI)-Child form, with Italian standardization [39]. The questionnaire features 29 items and 4 open-ended questions and includes four specific subscales, including Cognitive Self-Instruction, Problem-Solving, Distraction, and Seeking Social Support. The rating scores on a three-point Likert scale [0 = never (not at all), 1 = sometimes, or 2 = Often (a lot)] for the closed-items. Higher score on all subscales indicated better coping with pain. In addition, at the end of the questionnaire we added four open-ended questions with the stem *"When I hurt..."*: *"I do; I think; I wish; I ask."* The open-ended questions were then classified by cluster analysis.

Emotional Adjustment

The use of self-report and behavioral rating questionnaires is the most common way used in research and clinical practice. An alternative and seemingly underutilized assessment methodology, in research area but not in clinical setting, for tapping internalizing/externalizing symptoms independently of language and self-report is projective drawing.

The use of projective drawings as part of an overall test battery can be useful to help children overcome communication barriers, revealing internal conflicts and subconscious distress [40], thereby allowing researchers to discriminate between children who need additional well-being adjustment examination [41, 42].

Adjustment-related emotional well-being was conceptualized using DAP and DAF according to Koppitz [28, 29] and Corman [43-45], respectively, as part of the self-concept adaptive mode. Self-concept can indeed affect role functioning and interdependence and can be related to physical pain. Two primary methods of interpreting the children's drawings were adopted in this study. In this regard, we assumed that the combination of both methods would define an algorithm able to measure representations of the child's psychological functioning and to assess basic defense mechanisms (i.e., psychological adjustment).

The first method used for either projective technique, namely the "integrative drawing scoring system," was first developed by Failo, Beals-Erickson and Venuti [46] as a global approach to score all drawing and ranking features on a 0-4 Likert scale, where 0 indicates "negative representations," whereas 4 stands for "positive representations." The higher the score, the better adjusted the child's self-representation and family perception.

The second scoring method used for the DAF was developed by Tambelli, Zavattini, and Mossi [30]. It consists of 9 scales based on the characteristics of the family figures, the links between them and the activities they share in the drawing. Specifically, by analyzing omissions and additions, we managed to compare the real family with the family depicted in the drawing so as to determine the role of identifications and to rank the significance assigned to the characters depicted on three nominal scales (i.e., priority, size and importance), in accordance with Corman's concept of "valorization/devalorization."

The other scoring method for DAP, developed by Koppitz [28, 29], uses a total of 30 emotional indicators (EIs) as objective signs reflecting a child's worries or anxieties, with two or more of such indicators being highly suggestive of emotional problems. Lastly, we were able to classify the EIs according to their presumed underlying emotional symptom (i.e., impulsivity, insecurity/inadequacy, anxiety, shyness/timidity and anger/aggressiveness) using the emotional and behavioral scores proposed by Koppitz [28] and repurposed by Dağlioğlu, Deniz, and Kan [31],

Analysis Plan

The results were analyzed using the Statistical Package for the Social Science (SPSS, V.21.0). In light of the two main goals of this study, we planned two types of investigations: the first one focused exclusively on the clinical group, whereas the second one aimed to compare the clinical group with a healthy control group. Each group was assessed within itself for EIs.

Regarding the comparison between the clinical and the healthy group, given the number of the participants (N = 30 + 30) and because some cells had less than 5 values, the data were analyzed using non-parametric methods (i.e., Mann–Whitney U-test, Spearman's rho and Fisher's Exact test). To examine the emotional indicators and the object relations within the family system, both derivable from the drawings of the clinical and healthy group, we used a Chi-Square test in crosstabs. This approach allowed us to estimate the possible socio-demographic differences between the two samples and better understand sample comparability. The two groups were matched by age. Descriptive measures were computed for all relevant variables, and comparisons were made between the two groups.

The data analysis involved descriptive statistics and content analysis of the drawing themes. Data from the semi-structured interviews were linked to the themes of the drawings, scored independently by two raters, and processed through triangulation into quantitative scores.

The EIs included in the drawings were correlated with each other and analyzed through the Koppitz method [28, 29]. The two raters' EI scores were highly correlated (Cohen's Kappa = .80, $P < .05$). The indexes of object relationships were also correlated with each other and analyzed through the Tambelli, Zavattini, and Mossi method [30]. The Family Drawing Indexes had a good inter-rater agreement as well (Cohen's Kappa = .75, $P < .05$).

To plan the analysis within the clinical group, the data were first examined for skewness, kurtosis, outliers and normalcy (Shapiro-Wilk): no transformations were necessary as the distribution was normal for all dependent variables considered.

Descriptive statistics were followed by Pearson's bivariate analysis to identify any existing correlations between variables. A series of ANOVAs was performed to assess differences in self- and family-representations and coping strategies as well as to identify the differences between coping strategies and time since diagnosis, age at diagnosis, pain intensity (present and past), relapse, age groups and gender.

To test the predictive influence of the treatment phase, type of therapy and other important variables on prior pain experiences, a series of linear regression analyses were conducted. Other regressions were also performed to test the hypothesis that other psychosocial variables could influence the coping strategies and the EIs of well-being and adjustment.

Thematic content analysis [47] of open-ended questions left at the end of the PPCI questionnaire was also carried out to determine when the child was experiencing pain.

RESULTS

Sample Description

Thirty children and young adolescents, 18 males (60%) and 12 females (40%) between 7 and 14 years of age (M = 10.00, SD = 2.28), suffering from various forms of hematologic malignancies were enrolled in the study. These pediatric cancer patients were matched with a healthy control group of same-age peers (M = 9.84 SD = 1.44).

According to SES analysis, all parents and children in either group were middle class Caucasian (M = 37.98, SD = 14.43 *vs.* M = 42.88, SD = 14.34). Most of the parents had completed college or higher education. In contrast, the parental occupational status varied between the mothers and fathers and within groups. The number of siblings was almost the same for either group. Socio-demographic characteristics of parents and children are described in Table 1.

Table 1. Socio-demographic characteristics of parents and children of the two study groups

Socio-demographic characteristics of parents and children	Clinical group N = 30	Healthy group N = 30
Mother's age (M_{years}, SD)	42.07 (4.89)	47.17 (5.84)
Father's age (M_{years}, SD)	46.0 (5.49)	45.95 (4.78)
Mother's Education (%)		
• 5 years of schooling	0	0
• 8 years of schooling	5 (16.7)	1 (3.3)
• 13 years of schooling	12 (40)	14 (46.7)
• >13 years of schooling	13 (43.3)	11 (36.7)
• Not reported	0	4 (13.3)
Father's Education (%)		
• 5 years of schooling	1 (3.3)	0
• 8 years of schooling	7 (23.3)	3 (10)
• 13 years of schooling	10 (33.3)	13 (43.3)
• >13 years of schooling	10 (33.3)	9 (30)
• Not reported	2 (6.7)	5 (16.7)
Mother's Occupational status (%)		
• Househusband/unemployed	3 (10)	1 (3.3)
• Blue-collar workers	18 (60)	6 (20)
• Clerk/Freelancer	2 (6.7)	10 (33.3)
• Manager/Doctor	7 (23.3)	9 (30)
• Not reported	0	4 (13.3)
Father's Occupational status (%)		
• Househusband/unemployed	2 (6.7)	0
• Blue-collar workers	12 (40)	10 (33.3)
• Clerk/Freelancer	6 (20)	6 (20)
• Manager/Doctor	8 (26.7)	9 (30)
• Not reported	2 (6.7)	5 (16.7)
S.E.S (M_{years}, SD)	37.98 (14.43)	42.88 (14.34)
• Low – 10 thru 26.5 (%)	6 (20)	4 (13.3)
• Medium - 27 thru 44.5 (%)	15 (50)	11 (36.7)
• High - 45 thru hi (%)	9 (30)	12 (40)
• not calculable	0	3 (10)
No. Siblings (%)		
• 0	3 (10)	3 (10)
• 1	18 (60)	16 (53.3)
• ≥2	9 (30)	11 (36.7)

Table 1. (Continued)

Socio-demographic characteristics of parents and children	Clinical group N = 30	Healthy group N = 30
Child's Gender (%)		
• Male	18 (60)	14 (46.7)
• Female	12 (40)	16 (53.3)
Child's Age (M_{years}, SD)	10.00 (2.28)	9.84 (1.44)
• 7-10 years (%)	18 (60)	18 (60)
• 11-14 years (%)	12 (40)	12 (40)

Table 2. Medical characteristics of the clinical group patients

Medical characteristics	N = 30
Present pain (M, SD)	1.57 (2.06)
Past pain (M, SD)	6.53 (3.32)
Age at diagnosis (M_{month}, SD)	103.53 (34.20) range 44-140
Time since diagnosis (M_{month}, SD)	16.50 (16.83) range 2-55
Diagnosis (%)	
• acute lymphoblastic leukemia	23 (76.6)
• acute myeloid leukemia	3 (13.3)
• Hodgkin's lymphoma	2 (6.7)
• non-Hodgkin's lymphoma	1 (3.4)
Phase of treatment (%)	
• Induction	9 (30)
• Consolidation	4 (13.3)
• Re-induction	4 (13.3)
• Bone marrow transplant	4 (13.3)
• Maintenance	5 (16.7)
• Stop	4 (13.3)
Relapse (%)	
• Yes	4 (13.3)
• No	26 (86.7)
Concomitant psychosocial problems (%)	
• Yes	22 (73.3)
• No	8 (26.7)

In the clinical group, 86.7% (n = 26) of children had never faced a relapse. Furthermore, they could be grouped according to the following phases of treatment: induction (30%); consolidation (13.3%); re-induction (13.3%); bone marrow transplant (13.3%); maintenance (16.7%); and end of treatment (13.3%). Most of the children (73.3%) had concomitant psychosocial problems (e.g., another disease, a disease in the family, a death of close relatives or a recent divorce of parents).

The children in the clinical group reported low present pain intensity (M = 1.57, SD = 2.06), but their rating of prior pain (i.e., average of all pain during hospital stay) was moderate to severe (M = 6.53, SD = 3.32). The clinical characteristics of the pediatric cancer patients are described in Table 2.

Differences in Emotional Well-Being and Internalized System of Relations in Youth with Cancer Compared to Otherwise Healthy Children

This section reports the findings of the procedures conducted to determine the differences between the two study cohorts in terms of child's self-concept and family perception, with the latter being the prototype of the most intimate network of interconnected relationships a child has. For this purpose, we compared DAPs and DAFs from 30 pediatric cancer patients undergoing treatment with those from otherwise healthy children. All results are provided in tabular form.

During the entire interview and drawing process, most of the children showed a "collaborative/exploratory" behavior (73.3% in the clinical group and 86.7% in the healthy group). Only 26.7% of pediatric cancer patients and 13.3% of healthy kids adopted a "collaborative/non-exploratory" behavior, whereas none of them displayed a "resistant" or "refusing" behavior.

Children's Self-Perception of Well-Being through DAP

Concerning the general observations conducted during the drawing process and the answer provided by the children at the end of the process, we found a significantly higher number of corrections, in terms of erased areas, and stick figures, as opposed to an entire body, in the clinical *vs.* healthy group ($x^2 = 4.043$; $P = .044$ and $x^2 = 4.286$; $P = .038$, respectively). This index along with others (see the results below) tends to suggest under-use and anxiety surrounding the body [31]. See Table 3 for more details.

Table 3. Distribution of general observational characteristics in the study groups' DAPs

Observational characteristics	Clinical group N = 30	Healthy group N = 30	X^2	P
Who drew?			5.800	n.s.
• Himself/herself	2 (6.6)	8 (26.7)		
• Father/mother	6 (20)	2 (6.6)		
• Friends/siblings	11 (36.7)	9 (30)		
• Invented	11 (36.7)	11 (36.7)		
Excessive corrections			4.043	.044
• yes	6 (20)	1 (3.3)		
• no	24 (80)	29 (96.7)		
Age difference (with the real one)			2.411	n.s.
• yes	11 (36.7)	17 (56.7)		
• no	19 (63.3)	13 (43.3)		
More happy or sad?			1.964	n.s.
• happy	26 (86.7)	29 (96.7)		
• sad	4 (13.3)	1 (3.3)		
Stick figure			4.286	.038
• yes	4 (13.3)	0		
• no	26 (86.7)	30 (100)		

Table 4 reports the age and gender distribution of impulsivity-related characteristics in the children's DAPs. Of note, 26.7% of children in the clinical group and 6.7% in the healthy group omitted the neck in their human figure drawings ($P < .05$).

Table 5 shows that 16.7% of children in the clinical group did not complete the hands in their drawings (P = n.s.), whereas 13.3% of them drew tiny heads (P = n.s.). Despite the lack of statistical significance, it is important to point out that none of these indicators were present in the drawing of the children's belonging to the healthy group.

**Table 4. Distribution of impulsivity-related characteristics
in the study groups' DAPs**

Impulsivity	Clinical group		Healthy group	
	EI N	%	EI N	%
Poor body part integration	6	20	3	10
Gross limb asymmetry	2	6.7	4	13.3
Transparencies	1	3.3	-	-
Big figure	2	6.7	-	-
Neck omission*	8	26.7	2	6.7
Total of impulsivity indicators**	19	63.3	9	30

$*x^2 = 4.320; P = .040; **x^2 = 6.70; P < .001.$

**Table 5. Distribution of insecurity/inadequacy-related characteristics
in the study groups' DAPs**

Insecurity/inadequacy	Clinical group		Healthy group	
	EI N	%	EI N	%
Slanted figure	2	6.7	-	-
Tiny head	4	13.3	-	-
Omission of hands	-	-	-	-
Monster or grotesque figure	1	3.3	-	-
Omission of arms	-	-	-	-
Omission of legs	-	-	-	-
Omission of feet	-	-	-	-
Hands cut off	5	16.7	1	3.3
Total of insecurity/inadequacy indicators**	12	40	1	3.3

$**x^2 = 11.880; P < .001.$

As shown in Table 6, no statistical difference between the two study groups was found regarding anxiety EIs.

As can be inferred from Table 7, the omission of the nose, which is an indicator of shyness and timidity, occurred more frequently than other characteristics. Although no statistical difference was found, it is noteworthy to point out that the control group displayed more overall shyness/timidity EIs than the clinical group.

**Table 6. Distribution of anxiety-related characteristics
in the study groups' DAPs**

Anxiety	Clinical group			Healthy group		
	EI N		%	EI N		%
Shading of face	1		3.3	1		3.3
Shading of body or limbs	1		3.3	1		3.3
Shading of hands or neck	1		3.3	-		-
Legs pressed together	1		3.3	3		10
Omission of eyes	-		-	-		-
Omission of body	-		-	-		-
Three or more figures drawn[¥]	-		-	1		3.3
Total of anxiety indicators	4		13.2	6		19.9

[¥]Despite the lack of consensus on the interpretation of this indicator in previous studies, we chose to categorize it as an anxiety indicator.

**Table 7. Distribution of shyness/timidity-related
characteristics in the study groups' DAPs**

Shyness/Timidity	Clinical group			Healthy group		
	EI N		%	EI N		%
Tiny figure	3		10	4		13.3
Short arms	3		10	7		23.3
Arms clinging to body	-		-	2		6.7
Omission of nose	9		30	8		26.7
Omission of mouth	-		-	-		-
Total of shyness/timidity indicators	15		50	21		70

As shown in Table 8, no statistical difference between the two groups was found concerning anger EIs.

Of note, the frequency of EI occurrence in the drawings of the clinical *vs.* control group was higher (Mann-Whitney U = 336.500; *P* (exact 1 tail) = .042). Moreover, when we tested the same hypothesis using a global approach, we found significant differences for both formal-structural DAP coding (Mann-Whitney U = 303.000; *P* (exact 1 tail) = .009) and content-DAP coding (Mann-Whitney U = 279.500; *P* (exact 1 tail) = .003).

**Table 8. Distribution of anger-related characteristics
in the study groups' DAPs**

Anger	Clinical group		Healthy group	
	EI N	%	EI N	%
Crossed eyes	1	3.3	-	-
Presence of teeth	1	3.3	1	3.3
Long arms	2	6.6	2	6.7
Big hands	4	13.3	-	-
Genitals	-	-	-	-
Total of anger indicators	8	26.5	3	10

Children's Perception of the Family through DAF

Several factors need to be taken into account when assessing a child's perception of his/her family within the object relations theory concerning the family system. Most of the DAFs were similar to the DAPs in terms of pressure and types of strokes and lines used while drawing. With regard to the identification of desire, the response to the interview question: *"Who would you like to be?"* refers to a desire or tendency at the conscious level—that is to say that a child tends to choose the person best representing its "confessable" aspirations. Indeed, 40% of cancer patients and 43% of healthy children drew themselves together with parents or siblings as having the same sex as their own. This means that children are inclined to identify themselves with those family members "who represent the power, value and models that children would like to make their own" [32, p.33]. Thus, this important aspect highlights the sense of sexual belonging and the function it takes on in the organization of the Self. No statistical differences were found between the clinical and healthy group in this regard (see Table 9).

Comparing the actual composition of the families with those depicted in the drawings, we observed that 60% of sick children and 42.3% of healthy children drew their families without making changes.

In the remaining 40% of cases (56.7% in the healthy group), the changes consisted in omitting people, especially siblings (16.7% *vs.* 36.7% in the clinical and healthy group, respectively).

**Table 9. Distribution of "identification of desire"
in the study groups' DAFs**

Identification of desire	Clinical group		Healthy group	
	EI N	%	EI N	%
Self	12	40	13	43
Same-sex parent	3	10	7	23.3
No same-sex parent	1	3.3	-	-
Same-sex sibling	6	20	3	13.3
No same-sex sibling	3	10	1	3.3
Other/doesn't know	5	16.7	5	16.7

On the other hand, children without siblings added at least one brother or sister in 20% of cases (for both groups). The added figures, which like the omitted figures are here interpreted as different "identifications" of the subject rather than indicating unexpressed drives, are chiefly representative of children with whom there is a fraternal bond (20% for both groups).

No statistical differences were found between the clinical and healthy group (see Table 10).

As for the order (priority index) in which the family figures are drawn, the father often comes first in both groups (53.3% clinical group and 35.7% healthy group) (see Table 11, Priority). Assuming that there is a link between the emotional resonance of a family member and the size of that member's depiction, the father is also the most highly valorized figure in terms of height (79.3% clinical group and 60.7% healthy group), followed by the mother (24.8%) (see Table 11, Size).

Based on the number of attributes, the father is the figure who receives most attention among the sick children (58.6%). Conversely, the healthy children depicted themselves first (34.5%) and then the father (see Table 11, Importance).

**Table 10. Distribution of omitted and added figures
in the study groups' DAFs**

Omitted figures	Clinical group		Healthy group	
	N	%	N	%
Self	1	3.3	1	3.3
Mother	1	3.3	1	3.3
Father	-	-	2	6.7
Siblings	5 (24)	16.7	11 (27)	36.7
Nobody	23	76.7	15	50
Siblings	6	20	6	20
Other/animals	1	3.3	-	-
Nobody	23	76.7	24	80

**Table 11. Distribution of priority, size and importance
in the study groups' DAFs**

FD INDEXES	Clinical group N, (reference % within group)					Healthy group N, (reference % within group)				
	Self	Mother	Father	Sibling 1	Sibling 2	Self	Mother	Father	Sibling 1	Sibling 2
Priority	7 (24.1)	4 (14.3)	16 (53.3)	3 (15.8)	-	9 (31)	9 (31)	10 (35.7)	2 (11.8)	-
Size	1 (3.4)	5 (17.9)	23 (79.3)	-	-	2 (6.9)	7 (24.19)	17 (60.7)	-	2 (14.3)
Importance	5 (17.2)	4 (14.8)	17 (58.6)	2 (10)	-	10 (34.5)	5 (17.2)	9 (32.1)	1 (5.9)	-

FD = Family drawing.

According to the response given to the question *"Who is the happiest?"* and from the drawing observations, a difference between the clinical group was found, where the father is the least happy, compared to the control group ($x^2 = 7.68$; $P < .01$). A generally positive emotional tone was instead found for all the other characters (i.e., self, mother and siblings). From the question *"Who is the least happy"* no difference was observed between and within the 2 groups (see below Table 12).

Table 12. Distribution of the emotional tone
in the study groups' DAFs

FD INDEXES	Clinical group N, (reference % within group)						Healthy group N, (reference % within group)					
	Self	Mother	Father	Siblings	Everybody	Nobody	Self	Mother	Father	Sibling1	Everybody	Nobody
The happiest	6 (20)	8 (26.7)	1* (3.3)	8 (26.7)	4 (13.3)	3 (10)	6 (20)	5 (16.7)	9* (30)	6 (20)	2 (6.7)	2 (6.7)
The least happy	5 (16.7)	4 (13.3)	9 (30)	3 (10)	-	9 (30)	7 (23.3)	7 (23.3)	5 (16.7)	4 (13.3)	-	7 (23.3)

FD = Family drawing $*x^2 = 7.68$; $P < .01$.

Considering depicted closeness as an indicator of the dynamics of affections, we evaluated "where" children drew themselves with respect to other family members. Most of the sick children (51.7%) and 31% of healthy children placed themselves near at least one parent, followed by siblings (20.7% and 27.6%, respectively), thus emphasizing the bond of mutual understanding and liking that connects children with their parents and siblings (see Table 13).

Table 13. Distribution of closeness in the study groups' DAFs

Closeness	Clinical group (n=29)		Healthy group (n=28)	
	N	%	N	%
Mother	8	27.6	4	13.8
Father	7	24.1	5	17.2
Siblings	6	20.7	8	27.6
Other/animals	1	3.4	-	-
Between parents	1	3.4	5	17.2
Between siblings	2	6.9	1	3.4
Between siblings and parents	4	13.8	6	16.9

In conclusion, the comparison between the drawings of the clinical and control group through a global approach (formal DAF) showed an overall significant difference (Mann-Whitney U = 263.000; P (exact 1 tail) = .001).

Characterization of Pain-Coping Profiles and Emotional Well-Being Adjustments

We next sought to determine the pain-coping profiles adopted by pediatric cancer patients and their associations with pain intensity, disease, treatment procedures and family factors. As shown in Table 14, descriptive statistics analysis revealed that the most common coping style embraced by sick children was to seek social support.

Pearson's bivariate correlations were then computed between illness parameters, pain intensity, demographic variables, child and family dimensions and the pain-coping strategies developed by the children. Even though not all children's coping strategies were correlated with each other, cognitive self-instruction strategies were significantly correlated with those pertaining to problem solving (r =.409; $P = .025$) and social support (r =.508; $P = .004$). Furthermore, cognitive strategies were negatively correlated with parental SES (r = -.398; $P = .033$), while distraction strategies were negatively correlated with pain intensity at present time (r = -.398; $P = .029$).

From the thematic content analysis, four overarching themes were examined: *"What I do; What I think; What I wish;* and *What I ask."* The detailed description of the sub-themes contained in the children's writings is given below.

"What I Do That Helps Me When I Feel Pain"

Proactive behavior (n = 11; 36.7%): *"I play; I do a jigsaw; I draw what I like; I take a shower."* Passive behavior/alienation (n = 9; 30%): *"I do nothing; I cry and scream; I stay alone."* Seeking social support (n = 10; 33.3%): *"I play with mom and dad; I go to my mom and tell her that it hurts."*

"What I Think That Helps Me When I Feel Pain"

Fatalism (n = 10; 33.3%): *"It hurts and I can do nothing to stop it; The truth is that it hurts.";* Proactive behavior (n = 9; 30%): *"I could take some medicine to feel better; If I don't think I feel pain the aching will go away.";* Positive thinking (n = 11; 36.7%): *"I think of all my friends and having fun with them; I know I can make it; I think it does not really hurt that much."*

"What I Wish When I Feel Pain"

Healing (n = 20; 66.7%): *"I wish I felt better; I think I will heal soon; The pain will soon go away."* Consolation /distraction (n = 8; 13.3%): *"It would be nice to have a dog stay with me; I wish I could hang out with my friends; If only I could forget about it and just play";* Helplessness (n = 2; 6.7%): *"I have no hope; I don't want anybody to help me."*

"What I Ask That Helps Me When I Feel Pain"

Needing emotional closeness (n = 22; 73.3%): *"I ask my parents to stay close to me, and I like being cuddled by them; I ask if someone can stay with me and give me support."* Passive behavior (n = 4; 13.3%): *"I don't need anything; I ask if I can watch TV";* Some solutions (n = 4; 13.3%): *"I ask for medicine and cuddles; I ask how I can stop the pain."*

In the active phases of treatment (i.e., induction, consolidation, re-induction and bone marrow transplant), children reported that they had asked for more solutions than those sought after during non-active treatment (20% *vs.* 0%). They also stated that in the same period they had experienced a pattern of negativistic attitudes and passive resistance (30% *vs.* 0%).

Table 14. Descriptive statistics of children's pain-coping strategies

Coping Strategies	N	Mean	SD	Range
Seeking social support	30	7.63	3.26	2-13
Problem solving	30	6.47	2.93	1-13
Cognitive self-instruction	30	5.67	2.23	1-11
Distraction	30	5.30	3.03	1-12

An ANOVA was performed with the following dependent variables: time since diagnosis; age at diagnosis; pain intensity (present and past);

relapse; age group; and sex. The different coping strategies were included singularly as fixed factors.

There was a significant interaction between cognitive self-instruction strategies, age at diagnosis [$F(9,29) = 2.423$; $P = .048$] and gender [$F(9,29) = 2.578$; $P = .037$].

Another significant interaction was found between phase of therapy (active and maintenance) and problem solving [$F(10,19) = 3.537$; $P < .001$].

A linear regression model showed that cognitive self-instruction strategies were associated significantly with parental SES ($\beta = -.390$, $t = -2.243$, $P = .033$) (Table 15).

Furthermore, parental SES was also associated with the quality of parent's advice provided when the child was facing pain ($\beta = .382$, $t = 2.190$, $P = .037$) (Table 16).

Table 15. Linear regression analyses predicting cognitive self-instruction to deal with pain

| | Cognitive self-instruction to deal with pain | | | | |
	b (T)	SE b	β	R^2	ΔR^2
Constant	8.238	1.208		.152	.122
SES	-1.224	.546	*-.390**		

ΔR^2= change in R^2; β= standardized regression weights;*P < .05.

Table 16. Linear regression analyses predicting quality of parent's advice provided when the child had to face the pain

| | Quality of parent's advices provided when the child had to face the pain | | | | |
	b (T)	SE b	β	R^2	ΔR^2
Constant	1.476	.509		.146	.116
SES	.503	.230	*.382**		

ΔR^2= change in R^2; β= standardized regression weights;*P < .05.

As to other possible variables, we found that the age at diagnosis was correlated with pain intensity at present time ($r = .536$; $P = .002$). Furthermore, children currently participating in medical treatment therapy perceived different quality of parental advice when they had to face pain (r = -.382; *P* = .037), had a different ratings of prior pain (i.e., average of all pain during hospital stay) (r = -.382; *P* = .037), and made different choices regarding identification of desire (r = -.390; *P* = .033). The treatment phase was correlated with rating of prior pain (r = .363; *P* = .049).

A series of regression analyses measured the possible factors associated with prior pain (past). Results partially confirmed our hypothesis. With regard to prediction of level of prior pain, beta coefficients for the three predictors of past pain (average of all pain during hospital stay) were phase of treatment (β = .363, t = 1.147, *P* = .001), medical therapy (β = -.382, t = -2.189, *P* =.037) and real/invented DAF (β = .384, t = 2.162, *P* = .040) (Table 17).

Table 17. Linear regression analyses predicting rating of prior pain

	Rating of prior pain				
	b (T)	SE b	*β*	R^2	ΔR^2
Constant	4.490	1.147		.132	.101
phase of treatment	.652	.317	*.363**		
Constant	8.444	1.044		.146	.116
medical therapy (on/off)	-2.730	.1.147	*-.382**		
Constant	2.824	1.792		.148	.116
real/invented DAF	2.588	1.197	*.384**		

ΔR^2= change in R^2; β= standardized regression weights;*P < .05.

Next, we sought to determine the status of a child's psychological well-being in relation to its pain coping style. To this end, we assessed the children's inner awareness of their bodies, feelings and relationships through a global approach using the integrative scoring system in DAP and DAF.With respect to the self-representation drawings, DAP scores between formal coding and content coding were significantly and positively associated (r = 0.729; *P* < .001). In addition, the DAF scores, as indicators of family perception, were correlated with both formal and content DAP (r = .6027; *P* < .001; r = .527; *P* = .003, respectively). Importantly, the EI scores were correlated with all self-representation drawings: formal DAP (r = -.486; *P* = .006), content DAP (r = -.567; *P* = .001), attesting the *bona fide* of the two scoring methods. Moreover, the DAF scores were correlated with the type of behavioral attitude of the child during the treatment protocol (r = -.366; P = .047). Finally, we found a correlation between gender and formal DAP (r = -.554; $P < .001$), content DAP (r = .419; $P = .021$), DAF (r = -.594; $P < .001$) and EIs (r = .389; $P = .033$), whereas no significant correlations were found with child's age (Table 18).

Table 18. Descriptive statistics for the child's indicators of emotional well-being

Indicators of Emotional Well-Being	N	Mean	SD	Range
Formal DAP	30	2.23	.74	1-4
Content DAP	30	2.57	.85	1-4
Formal DAF	30	2.17	.69	1-4
Koppitz EIs	30	2.03	1.67	0-6

Through ANOVA, we assessed potential differences in self- and family-representations and coping strategies. There was a significant interaction between formal DAF and cognitive strategies [F(9,29) = 2.425, $P = .047$], as well as between problem solving strategies and content and formal DAP [F(11,29) = 2.472, $P = .043$; F(11,29) = 3.078, $P = .017$, respectively].

A series of hierarchical multiple regression analyses were conducted to examine whether variables such as gender, age and the various coping strategies from the four subscales of the PPCI questionnaire or from the open-ended questions could significantly predict the EIs. One of our models was able to identify a significant association between the number of indicators of emotional symptoms and the independent variables "gender" (step one) and "gender" and "type of thoughts when the child experiences pain" (step two). The best model was the second one [R 0 .558, $R^2 = .260$, F(1,29)= 6.095; $P = .019$, R^2 change = .260], indicating that gender ($\beta = .376$, t = -2.355, $P = .026$) and type of thoughts when the child has pain ($\beta = .400$, t = -2.500, $P = .019$) were the best factors associated with EIs (Table 19).

**Table 19. Hierarchical regression analyses predicting the
number of indicators of emotional symptoms**

	No. of indicators underlying emotional symptoms				
	b (T)	SE b	β	R^2	ΔR^2
Step 1				.152	.121
Constant	1.250	.452			
Gender	.670	.584	.389*		
Step 2				.311	.260
Constant	-.320	.753			
Gender	1.262	.536	.376*		
Type of thoughts when the child has pain	.785	.314	.400*		

ΔR^2= change in R^2; β= standardized regression weights;*P < .05.

CONCLUSION

In this study, our primary goal was to determine whether human figure
drawings depicted by children with cancer would be different from those
of healthy children in terms of Koppitz EIs—originally classified in 5
categories [28, 29] and recently revised by Dağlioğlu, Deniz, and Kan
[31]—and whether these differences would be predictive of difficulties in
long-term adaptation to pain.

In the impulsivity and insecurity/inadequacy categories, the total
number of EIs was significantly higher in children with cancer compared
to that of healthy children (63.3% *vs.* 30%; 40% *vs.* 3.3%, respectively), in
good agreement with results from a previous study using the same tools
[47]. This means that children with a serious disease tend to show a more
unstable behavior and are often unable to postpone their immediate needs
and impulses. Our findings are also in line with a study by Pinheiro et al.,
[48] showing how a change in self-image can be very stressful for children
and adolescents, making them feel completely inadequate because they
look different from their peers. Furthermore, insecurity in ill children arises
from the fear of being abandoned by their parents upon hospitalization or
from not knowing exactly their medical condition and the medical
procedures they will have to undergo [48].

With regard to the anger category, the differences in EIs between sick and healthy children were not statistically significant. This is not surprising as aggressive behaviors are commonly found especially in adolescents and occur more frequently against nurses. Such behaviors are not always apparent externally, but they become more obvious during unpleasant examinations, limitations, restrictions, blood transfusions and chemotherapy [48].

Moreover, in both groups we found low levels of anxiety and high levels of shyness/timidity, which is a trait associated with feelings of apprehension, lack of confidence and awkwardness. Timidity is highly related to low self-perception, such as low self self-esteem and insecurity, and it may indicate withdrawal or depression. Thus, while in healthy children timidity/shyness could be simply explained as a natural consequence of experiencing a new situation (e.g., being in contact with unfamiliar people such as hospital staff and researchers), in sick children it may instead indicate withdrawal or depression.

These results are in keeping with a previous study assessing physical self-concept, anxiety, depression and self-esteem in children with cancer *vs.* healthy children, with self-esteem and physical self-concept being the best predictors of depression and anxiety, respectively [49].

Although the levels of anxiety observed in our clinical group may seem surprisingly low, they are consistent with a large body of empirical literature indicating that young cancer patients often display levels of anxiety symptoms similar to those of their healthy peers or normative groups with subclinical or clinical levels of anxiety early after diagnosis. However, anxiety levels appear to revert to expected levels after 6-12 months of diagnosis [50, 51]. In addition, long-term pediatric cancer survivors did not show higher prevalence of anxiety compared to healthy children [52].

Taken together, our findings are in good agreement with those by Pinquart and co-workers reporting moderate to high levels of internalizing, but not externalizing, symptoms in children with cancer *vs.* healthy children [53].

Besides providing individual indicators of internal distress [54], family drawings can offer "narrative constructions" of relevant relationships in their utmost unconscious aspects, within the regulating emotions of the internal models [55]. Indeed, the relationships between feeling pain and reporting pain are highly context-dependent and central among those factors relevant to the experience of pain, family and culture [47, 56]. In line with these considerations, our data confirm that there are differences between the family drawings of sick *vs.* healthy children, both in terms of specific markers and global evaluation. The differences lie especially in the ways the paternal figure is being depicted, which is generally characterized by greater importance, size and priority compared to the other figures of the family, especially in children with cancer. Furthermore, in contrast to the clinical group, the father of a healthy child is clearly represented as the happiest person of the family.

Regarding the actual composition of the family, it is important to point out that 60% of children from either group drew the family making changes, which could be viewed as a self-defense mechanism based on repressing impulsive thoughts or insecurity feelings concerning the relationship with their parents. Such repressive behavior might be a consequence of the family reaction towards the child's internalized problems, which may vary in either group. A "repressive adaptive style" can be a pathway to resilience in children with cancer since an adaptive style is a much stronger predictor of psychosocial outcomes [57]. However, caution should be exercised when attributing psychological defense mechanisms before examining the specific case history of a child and its family.

We were able to partially address the aforementioned issue in the second part of our study, where we attempted to characterize the pain-coping profiles and emotional adjustments in our pediatric cancer patients. Indeed, we found a strong correlation between parental SES and quality of parental support: the higher the parental SES, the higher the quality of the parental advice provided to sick children. These results are in keeping with previous studies showing that sick children from families with lesser social and economic resources are at increased risk of maladjustment to pain [58].

In addition, we show that to a lower SES corresponds a greater "search for cognitive self-instruction to deal with pain." from the child's perspective, This finding differs from that of previous studies showing that uneducated parents with lower health literacy generally struggle to understand their child's treatment and side effects, most likely perceiving him/her as more vulnerable [57, 58].

Overall, consistent with past research [26, 60]), we show that parent coping-promoting behaviors (i.e., quality of parental advice provided to kids facing pain) are associated with higher rates of children's pain-coping profiles, such as cognitive self-instruction. Furthermore, our findings indicate that the main factors influencing pain self-ratings—estimated as the average of all pain during hospitalization—are represented by the various phases of treatment (e.g.., active *vs.* inactive therapy status) and by the presence of additions and/or omissions in family figure drawings.

Another important consideration to be made is that the total score of the indicators underlying emotional symptoms depends on the variables "gender" and "type of thoughts the child had when feeling pain." For example, girls dealing with pain tend to have more fatalistic thoughts than boys, which indicates a greater emotional distress in girls *vs.* boys. Overall, "seeking social support" seems to be the most effective strategy adopted by sick children to cope with pain, confirming findings from a previous survey on a similar Italian population [41].

Our study has some limitations that should be taken into account when interpreting our findings in view of future research on this topic.

First, our study was a convenience sampling survey with a relatively small sample size. In this regard, we performed a priori sample size calculation by GPower 3.1.9.2 [61], which determined that a sample size of 30 would be required to detect a medium effect size ($d = .50$) with an analysis of variance ($\alpha = .05$, power $= .60$). Thus, it appears that a larger sample size would have increased the strength of our analysis.

Second, in keeping with previous work examining the role of parental behavior in school-age children [62, 63], we have only measured dyadic interactions during episodes of pain (i.e., parent acceptance of a child's emotion during painful episodes and quality of parent's advices supplied to the child) during the whole observational period but not at a specific point in time. This may have caused biased interpretations, that is to say a tendency to interpret some situations in a too positive or too negative fashion. Furthermore, we only studied the child's own coping profiles but not the parental ones. It would have indeed been useful to address the parents' behaviors toward their sick child or explore their psychological reactions to caring for their own child, given the effect that parent functioning has on a child's adjustment to chronic pain [64]. It would have also been more informative to address the relationship between family functioning and child acute pain, including pain ratings, coping and parent-child interaction [65]. In this regard, the impact of family and cultural beliefs on children learning how to react to pain has been mainly investigated in primary school-age children [66, 67].

In conclusion, our mix-method approach has allowed us to perform an accurate assessment of the pain-coping process of pediatric cancer patients as it takes into account many variables that could not be otherwise investigated by a single tool and within one single psychological paradigm.

By complementing different theoretical constructions, this study demonstrates that many factors play a key role in the interplay between conscious and unconscious activations of a child's well-being. This information is then crucial for early identification of those kids at risk of developing maladjustments to cancer-related pain, for whom psychosocial intervention as well as focused parental support should be promptly initiated.

Funding Details and Acknowledgements

At the time the project was being implemented, Alessandro Failo was supported by a Doctoral Scholarship from the University of Trento with the main grant from Fondazione Trentina per la Ricerca sui Tumori (FTRT). We thank all the healthcare professionals who helped us during this project. We would like to thank the many children and parents who participated in the study.

REFERENCES

[1] Ward, Elizabeth, Carol DeSantis, Anthony Robbins, Betsy Kohler, and Ahmedin Jemal. 2014. "Childhood and Adolescent Cancer Statistics, 2014." *CA: A Cancer Journal for Clinicians* 64:83-103. doi:10.3322/caac.21219.

[2] Imbach, Paul, Thomas Kühne, and Robert J. Arceci. 2006. *Pediatric oncology: a comprehensive guide.* Berlin: Springer.

[3] Pizzo, Philips A., and Poplack David G. 2016. *Principles and Practice of Pediatric Oncology.* 7th ed. Philadelphia: Wolters Kluwer.

[4] Cox, Lauren E., Ansley E. Kenney, Jennifer L. Harman, Niki Jurbergs, Andrew E. Molnar, and Victoria W. Willard. 2019. "Psychosocial Functioning of Young Children Treated for Cancer: Findings From a Clinical Sample." *Journal of Pediatric Oncology Nursing* 36:17-23. doi: 10.1177/1043454218813905.

[5] Darcy, Laura, Susanne Knutsson, Karina Huus, Karin Enskär. 2014. "The everyday life of the young child shortly after receiving a cancer diagnosis, from both children's and parent's perspectives." *Cancer Nursing* 37:445-456. doi: 10.1097/NCC.0000000000000114.

[6] Ganjavi, Anahita, Ali Reza Abedin, and Nader Monirpoor. 2010. "Predicting Factors of Adjustment in Iranian Children with Cancer." *Procedia Social and Behavioral Sciences* 5:859-864.

[7] Williams, Lauren K., Karen E. Lamb, and Maria C. McCarthy. 2014. "Behavioral Side Effects of Pediatric Acute Lymphoblastic Leukemia Treatment: The Role of Parenting Strategies." *Pediatric Blood & Cancer* 61:2065-2070. https://doi.org/0.1002/pbc.25164.

[8] Lee, Mei-Yin, Pei-Fan Mu, Shwu-Feng Tsay, Shin-Shang Chou, Yu-Chih Chen, and Tai-Tong Wong. 2012. "Body Image of Children and Adolescents with Cancer: A Metasynthesis on Qualitative Research Findings." *Nursing & Health Sciences* 14:381–90. doi:10.1111/j.1442-2018.2012.00695.x.

[9]   Sloper, Patricia. 2000. "Predictors of distress in parents of children with cancer: A prospective study." *Journal of Pediatric Psychology*, 25:79-91. https://doi.org/10.1093/jpepsy/25.2.79.

[10]   Sint Nicolaas, Simone, Peter Hoogerbrugge, Esther Bergh, José Custers, Sofia Gameiro, Reinoud Gemke, Chris Verhaak, et al. 2016. "Predicting Trajectories of Behavioral Adjustment in Children Diagnosed with Acute Lymphoblastic Leukemia." *Supportive Care in Cancer* 24:4503–13. doi:10.1007/s00520-016-3289-9.

[11]   Vlachioti, Efrosini, Pantelis Perdikaris, Efstathia Megapanou, Floria Sava, and Vasiliki Matziou. 2016. "Assessment of Quality of Life in Adolescent Patients with Cancer and Adolescent Survivors of Childhood Cancer." *Journal for Specialists in Pediatric Nursing* 21:178–88. doi:10.1111/jspn.12154.

[12]   Rudolph, Karen D., Marie D. Dennig, and John R. Weisz. 1995. "Determinants and Consequences of Children's Coping in the Medical Setting: Conceptualization, Review, and Critique." *Psychological Bulletin* 118:328–57. doi:10.1037/0033-2909.118.3.328.

[13]   Collins, John J., Michael M. Stevens, Charles B. Berde. 2008. "Pediatric cancer pain." In *Cancer Pain*. 2th ed, edited by Nigel Sykes, Michael Bennet, Chun-su Yuan, 345-358. London: Hodder & Stroughton press.

[14]   Moody, Karen, Marc Meyer, Carol A. Mancuso, Mary Charlson, and Laura Robbins. "Exploring Concerns of Children with Cancer." *Supportive Care In Cancer* 14:960–66. doi:10.1007/s00520 -006-0024-y.

[15]   Collins, John J., Tom D. Devine, Gina S. Dick, Elizabeth A. Johnson, Henry A. Kilham, C. Ross Pinkerton, M. M. Stevens, Howard T. Thaler, and Russell K. Portenoy. 2002. "The Measurement of Symptoms in Young Children with Cancer: The Validation of the Memorial Symptom Assessment Scale in Children Aged 7-12." *Journal of Pain and Symptom Management*, 23:10-16.

[16]   Cline, Rebecca J. W., Felicity W. K. Harper, Louis A. Penner, Amy M. Peterson, Jeffrey W. Taub, and Terrance L. Albrecht. 2006.

"Parent Communication and Child Pain and Distress during Painful Pediatric Cancer Treatments." *Social Science & Medicine* 65:883-898. doi:10.1016/j.socscimed.2006.03.007.

[17] Hedström, Mariann, Kristina Haglund, Mariann I. Skolin, Louise von Essen. 2003. "Distressing Events for Children and Adolescents with Cancer: Child, Parent, and Nurse Perceptions." *Journal of Pediatric Oncology Nursing* 20:120-132. doi: 10.1053/jpon.2003.76.

[18] Twycross, Alison, Roslyn Parker, Anna Williams, and Faith Gibson. 2015. "Cancer-Related Pain and Pain Management: Sources, Prevalence, and the Experiences of Children and Parents." *Journal of Pediatric Oncology Nursing* 32:369-384. doi: 10.1177/1043454214563751.

[19] Menossi, Maria José, Regina A. G. Lima, Adriana Kátia Corrêa. 2008. Pain in children and adolescents with cancer. *Rev Latino-am Enfermagem* 16:489-494. http://producao.usp.br/handle/BDPI/3472.

[20] Duffy, Elizabeth A., Nancy Dias, Verna Hendricks-Ferguson, Melody Hellsten, Micah Skeens-Borland, Cliff Thornton, and Lauri A. Linder. 2019. "Perspectives on Cancer Pain Assessment and Management in Children." *Seminars in Oncology Nursing* 35:261-273. https://doi.org/10.1016/j.soncn.2019.04.007.

[21] Thorsell-Cederberg J., Dahl J., von Essen L., and Ljungman G. 2017. "An Acceptance-Based Intervention for Children and Adolescents with Cancer Experiencing Acute Pain – a Single-Subject Study." *Journal of Pain Research* 10: 2195-2203. http://dx.doi.org/10.2147/JPR.S139087.

[22] Schechter, Neil L., Charles B. Berde, Myron-Yaster Berde. 2003. *Pain in infants, children and adolescents.* 2th ed. Philadelphia: Lippincott Williams & Wilkins.

[23] Watson, David, Anna Clark, and Auke Tellegen. 1988. "Development and Validation of Brief Measures of Positive and Negative Affect: The PANAS Scales." *Journal of Personality and Social Psychology* 54:1063-1070. http://dx.doi.org/10.1037/0022-3514.54.6.1063.

[24] Compas, Bruce E., Jennifer K. Connor-Smith, Heidi Saltzman, Alexandra Harding Thomsen, and Martha E Wadsworth. 2001. "Coping with Stress during Childhood and Adolescence : Problems, Progress, and Potential in Theory and Research." *Psychological Bulletin* 127:87-127. doi:10.1037//0033-2909.127.1.87.

[25] Caes, Line, Liesbet Goubert, Patricia Devos, Joris Verlooy, Yves Benoit, and Tine Vervoort. 2014. "The Relationship Between Parental Catastrophizing About Child Pain and Distress in Response to Medical Procedures in the Context of Childhood Cancer Treatment: A Longitudinal Analysis." *Journal of Pediatric Psychology* 39:677-686. doi:10.1093/jpepsy/jsu034.

[26] Spagrud, Lara J., Carl L. Von Baeyer, Kaiser Ali, Christopher Mpofu, Louise Penkman Fennell, Kaethie Friesen, and Jan Mitchell. 2008. "Pain, Distress, and Adult-Child Interaction during Venipuncture in Pediatric Oncology : An Examination of Three Types of Venous Access." *Journal of Pain and Symptom Management* 36:173-184. doi:10.1016/j.jpainsymman.2007.10.009.

[27] Orbuch, Terri L., Carla Parry, Mark Chesler, Jennifer Fritz, and Paula Repetto. 2005. "Parent-Child Relationships and Quality of Life: Resilience among Childhood Cancer Survivors." *Family Relations* 54:171–183. http://dx.doi.org/10.1111/j.0197-6664.2005.00014.x.

[28] Koppitz, Elizabeth M. 1966. "Emotional indicators on human figure drawings and school achievement of first and second graders." *Journal of Clinical Psychology* 22:481-483. https://doi.org/10.1002/1097-4679(196610)22:4<481::AID-JCLP2270220436>3.0.CO;2-D.

[29] Koppitz, Elizabeth, M. 1983 *Psychological evaluation of human figure drawings by middle school pupils.* London: Grune & Stratton.

[30] Tambelli Renata, Zavattini Giulio C., Mossi Piergiorgio. 1995 *[The sense of family] Il senso della famiglia. Le relazioni affettive del bambino nel "Disegno della famiglia."* Roma: Nuova Italia Scientifica.

[31] Dağlioğlu, H. Elif, Ümit Deniz, and Adnan Kan. 2010. "A Study on the Emotional Indicators in 5-6 Year-Old Girls' and Boys' Human

Figure Drawings." *Procedia Social and Behavioral Sciences* 2:1503-1510. https://doi.org/10.1016/j.sbspro.2010.03.226.

[32] Dolidze, Khatuna, Emma L. Smith, and Kate Tchanturia. 2013. "A Clinical Tool for Evaluating Emotional Well-Being: Self-Drawings of Hospitalized Children." *Journal of Pediatric Nursing* 28:470-478. doi: 10.1016/j.pedn.2013.02.026.

[33] Dutta, Moon Moon, and Nilanjana Sanyal. 2016. "A Comparative Study of Emotional Characteristics of Children with and without ADHD by 'Draw a Man Test.'" *SIS Journal of Projective Psychology & Mental Health* 23:27-33. ISSN:0971-6610.

[34] Hollingshead, August B. 1975. *Four-factor index of social status.* New Haven, CT: Yale University unpublished manuscript.

[35] Bornstein, Marc H., Chun-Shin Hahn, Joan T. D. Suwalsky, and O. Maurice Haynes. 2003. "Socioeconomic Status, Parenting, and Child Development: The Hollingshead Four-Factor Index of Social Status and The Socioeconomic Index of Occupations." In *Socioeconomic Status, Parenting, and Child Development.*, edited by Marc H. Bornstein and Robert H. Bradley, 29–82. Monographs in Parenting Series. Mahwah, NJ: Lawrence Erlbaum Associates.

[36] von Baeyer, Carl L. 2009. "Children's self-report of pain intensity: what we know, where we are headed." *Pain research & management* 14:39-45. doi:10.1155/2009/259759.

[37] Mathews, Brittany L. 2012. "The relationship of attachment, maternal emotional socialization, and maternal coping with social anxiety during adolescence." MA diss., Kent State University.

[38] Roberti, Lorenzo. 2014. [*Draw-a-Family Test in a clinical field*] *Il Disegno della Famiglia in ambito Clinico e Giuridico Peritale. Guida pratica all'interpretazione.* Milano: Franco Angeli.

[39] Bonichini, Sabrina, and Giovanna Axia. 2000. "[Evaluation of pain coping strategies in school-age children] La valutazione delle strategie di coping al dolore fisico nei bambini di età scolare." *Psicologia Clinica dello Sviluppo* 1:97-124. doi:10.1449/586.

[40] Hatano, Yutaka, Miwa Yamada, Kanae Nakagawa, Hiromi Nanri, Masatoshi Kawase, and Kenji Fukui. 2014. "Using Drawing Tests to

Explore the Multidimensional Psychological Aspects of Children with Cancer." *Japanese Journal of Clinical Oncology* 44:1009-1012. doi:10.1093/jjco/hyu116.

[41] Tielsch, Anna H., and Patricia Jackson Allen. 2005. "Listen to Them Draw: Screening Children in Primary Care through the Use of Human Figure Drawings." *Pediatric Nursing* 31:320-27. ISSN:0097-9805.

[42] Waweru, Sylvia M., Annette Reynolds, and Ellen B. Buckner. 2008. "Perceptions of Children with HIV/AIDS from the USA and Kenya: Self-Concept and Emotional Indicators." *Pediatric Nursing* 34:117–24. PMID: 18543836.

[43] Corman, Louis. 1964. *[The family drawing test] Le test du dessin de famille*. Paris: Presses Universitaires de France.

[44] Corman, Louis. 1965. "The family drawing test: significance of added persons." *Rev Neuropsychiatr Infant* 13:67-81. PMID: 14268093.

[45] Corman, Louis. 1967. "The double in the family-drawing test: its psychopathological significance." *L' Evolution Psychiatrique* 32:117-147. PMID: 4875863.

[46] Failo, Alessandro, Paola Venuti, Sarah Beals-Erickson. 2018. "Coping strategies and emotional well-being in children with disease-related pain." *Journal of Child Health Care* 22:84-96. doi:10.1177/1367493517749326.

[47] Kortesluoma, Riitta-Liisa. 2009. "Hospitalized children as social actors in the assessment and management of their pain." PhD diss., University of Oulu.

[48] Pinheiro, Iracema do Vale, Allyson Guimarães da C., Débora C B Rodrigues, Nália de P. Oliveira, Adriana Malheiro, and Josafá L Ramos. 2015. "Hospital Psychological Assessment with the Drawing of the Human Figure: A Contribution to the Care to Oncologic Children and Teenagers." *Psychology* 6:484-500. doi: 10.4236/jsbs.2012.24020.

[49] Bragado, Carmen, M., José Hernández-Lloreda, Luisa Sánchez-Bernardos, and Susana Urbano. 2008. Physical self-concept, anxiety,

depression, and self-esteem in children with cancer and healthy children without cancer history. *Psicothema* 20:413-19.

[50] Katz, Lynn Fainsilber, Kaitlyn Fladeboe, Kevin King, Kyrill Gurtovenko, Joy Kawamura, Debra Friedman, Bruce Compas, et al. 2018. "Trajectories of Child and Caregiver Psychological Adjustment in Families of Children with Cancer." *Health Psychology* 37:725–35. doi:10.1037/hea0000619.supp.

[51] Myers, Regina M., Lyn Balsamo, Xiaomin Lu, Meenakshi Devidas, Stephen P. Hunger, William L. Carroll, Naomi J. Winick, Kelly W. Maloney, and Nina S. Kadan-Lottick. 2014. A prospective study of anxiety, depression, and behavioral changes in the first year after a diagnosis of childhood acute lymphoblastic leukemia. *Cancer*, 120:1417-1425. http://dx.doi.org/10.1002/cncr.28578.

[52] Wogelius, Pia, Steen Rosthøj, Göran Dahllöf, and Sven Poulsen. 2009. "Dental Anxiety among Survivors of Childhood Cancer: A Cross-Sectional Study." *International Journal of Paediatric Dentistry* 19:121-126. doi:10.1111/j.1365-263X.2008.00944.x.

[53] Pinquart, Martin, and Yuhui Shen. 2011. Behavior problems in children and adolescents with chronic physical illness: A meta-analysis. *Journal of Pediatric Psychology* 36:1003-1016. doi:10. 1093/jpepsy/jsq104.

[54] Goldner, Limor, and Miri Scharf. 2011. "Children's Family Drawings: A Study of Attachment, Personality, and Adjustment." *Art Therapy: Journal of the American Art Therapy Association* 28:11-18. http://dx.doi.org/10.1080/07421656.2011.557350.

[55] De Coro, Alessandra, Renata Tambelli, and Marco Cundari. 2008." [Drawn-A-Family. Relationship between parents and children by drawing's analysis] Il disegno della famiglia. Le relazioni tra genitori e figli attraverso l'analisi del disegno." In: [*Guidelines in testology*] *Linee di ricerca in testologia*, edited by Franco Del Corno, Margherita Lang, 415-470. Milano: Franco Angeli.

[56] Stevens, Bonnie, M. Hunsberger and G. Browne 1987. "Pain in Children: Theoretical, Research, and Practice Dilemmas." *Journal of Pediatric Nursing* 2:154-166. PMID: 3648121.

[57] Phipps, Sean. 2007. "Adaptive Style in Children with Cancer: Implications for a Positive Psychology Approach." *Journal of Pediatric Psychology* 9: 1055-1066. doi:10.1093/jpepsy/jsm060.

[58] Ryan, Jamie L., Angelica R. Eddington, Stephanie E. Hullmann, Rachelle R. Ramsey, Cortney Wolfe-Christensen, John M. Chaney, and Larry L. Mullins. 2013. "An Examination of Parenting Capacity Variables and Child Adjustment Outcomes Across Socioeconomic Level in Pediatric Cancer." *Children's Health Care* 42:281–93. doi:10.1080/02739615.2013.816617.

[59] Sanders, Lee M., Valerie T. Thompson, James D. Wilkinson. 2007. "Caregiver Health Literacy and the Use of Child Health Services." *Pediatrics* 119:e86-92. doi:10.1542/peds.2005-1738.

[60] Blount, Ronald L, Tiina Piira, Lindsey L Cohen, Patricia S Cheng, and Kenneth J Tarnowski. 2006. "Pediatric Procedural Pain." *Behavior Modification in Pediatric Settings*, 30:24-49. doi: 0.1177/0145445505282438.

[61] Faul, Franz, Edgar Erdfelder, Albert-Georg Lang, and Axel Buchner. 2007. "G*Power 3: A Flexible Statistical Power Analysis Program for the Social, Behavioral, and Biomedical Sciences." *Behavior Research Methods* 39:175–91. doi:10.3758/BF03193146.

[62] Boerner, Katelynn E., Kathryn A. Birnie, Line Caes, Meghan Schinkel, and Christine T. Chambers. 2014. "Sex Differences in Experimental Pain among Healthy Children: A Systematic Review and Meta-Analysis." *Pain* 155:983-993. doi: 10.1016/j.pain. 2014.01.031.

[63] Chambers, Christine. 2003. "The role of family factors in pediatric pain." In: *Pediatric pain: biological and social context*, edited by Patrick J McGrath, and Allen Finley, 99-130. Seattle: IASP Press.

[64] Palermo, Tonia M., and Eccleston Christopher. 2009. "Parents of children and adolescents with chronic pain." *Pain* 146:15-17. doi: 10.1016/j.pain.2009.05.009.

[65] Birnie, Kathryn A., Christine T. Chambers, Jill Chorney, Conrad V. Fernandez, Patrick J. McGrath, and Cynthia A. Gerhardt, Cynthia A. Berg, Deborah J. Wiebe and Grayson N. Holmbeck Guest Editors.

2017. "A Multi-Informant Multi-Method Investigation of Family Functioning and Parent-Child Coping during Children's Acute Pain." *Journal of Pediatric Psychology* 42:28-39. https://doi.org/10.1093/jpepsy/jsw045.

[66] Azize, Pary M., Ann Humphreys, and Allegra Cattani. 2011. "The Impact of Language on the Expression and Assessment of Pain in Children." *Intensive & Critical Care Nursing* 27:235-243. doi: 10.1016/j.iccn.2011.07.002.

[67] Fortier, Michelle A., Antonio M. Del Rosario, Abraham Rosenbaum, and Zeev N. Kain. 2010. "Beyond Pain: Predictors of Postoperative Maladaptive Behavior Change in Children." *Pediatric Anesthesia* 20:445–53. doi:10.1111/j.1460-9592.2010.03281.x.

In: Coping with Chronic Illness   ISBN: 978-1-53616-775-7
Editor: Meghan Mendoza   © 2020 Nova Science Publishers, Inc.

Chapter 3

CHILDREN'S COPING WITH CHRONIC ILLNESS: REDUCING ANXIETY AND RECOGNIZING RESILIENCE

L. A. Nabors and S. M. Gomes*

Health Promotion and Education Program, School of Human Services,
College of Education, Criminal Justice, and Human Services,
University of Cincinnati, Cincinnati, Ohio, US

ABSTRACT

Due to medical advances, more children with chronic illnesses are facing medical procedures. Many of them need assistance learning to cope with medical procedures and extended hospital stays. This chapter provides information on anxiety and worry management strategies for children with chronic illnesses. An emphasis on developing strategies based on the child's existing coping strategies can ensure that strategies will be used in stressful situations and during hospital procedures. Moreover, children with chronic illnesses may be resilient and find hope in many things, so positive aspects of child coping will be presented in this chapter. Additionally, conceptualizing coping as a family affair can be critical to ensuring that the child receives the support he or she needs.

* Corresponding Author's E-mail: naborsla@ucmail.uc.edu.

Siblings can be critical supports if the child faces an extended hospital stay and siblings are able to stay nearby. Ensuring that the family is coping well, can translate to improved coping for the child and the parent who is with the child, if an extended hospital stay is needed. Children with chronic illnesses and their families may be marked by resilience and a search for meaning and positive functioning as they strive to cope with a difficult family stressor. Thus, strategies for encouraging family coping efforts and resilience also will be a focus of discussion in this chapter. Future research needs to continue to focus on helping the child cope with stress and worry, related to their conditions and medical procedures. At the same time, recording instances of hope and resilience provides a strengths-based approach that can guide ideas for improving family coping and, ultimately, child coping.

Keywords: chronic illness, children, families, coping, resilience

INTRODUCTION

Approximately 10 million children and adolescents in the United States have been diagnosed with a chronic illness (Algozzine and Ysseldyke 2006). Chronic illnesses are defined as, "…illnesses or impairments that are expected to last for an extended period of time and require medical attention and care that is beyond what is normally expected for an individual of the same age" (p. 18; Ollendick, and Schroeder 2003). Between 15% and 19% of children in the United States lives with at least one chronic illness (Churchill et al. 2010; Martire and Hegelson 2017), with as many as 20% of children living with a chronic illness experiencing illness-related impairments (Bethell et al. 2011). Due to improved medical treatment, this number is increasing in tandem with the increase in survival rate for these children (Compas et al. 2012). The increase in lifespan for children with pediatric chronic illness has also led to a rise in the number of medical procedures that children face throughout life. The consequences of the illness, as well as increased procedures, are associated with more negative impact including stress, anxiety, pain, and have emotional and social implications (Compas et al. 2012).

When coping with their illnesses, children and adolescents with chronic illnesses may encounter painful procedures and recurring hospitalizations, loneliness and social and peer isolation (especially when in the hospital), school absences, and difficult, restrictive treatment regimens. Pinquart (2013) noted that it is important to promote resilience in youth with chronic illnesses as they may face low self-esteem related to the issues they face because of their illnesses. This population must manage symptoms that lead to physical and lifestyle changes, including restricted or partial participation in school and sports, as well as limitations related to invasive treatments, pain, and illness symptoms, which can change the nature of their involvement in daily activities (Bethell et al. 2011; Trowbridge and Mische-Lawson 2014). Furthermore, childhood spontaneity may be restrained due to physical changes or pain, leading to challenges with social relationships and concerns regarding the future and health (Gannoni and Shute 2010). Children with chronic illnesses may face limited social opportunities, both from decreases in their abilities to participate in extracurricular activities and constraints in their time to form friendships (Compas et al. 2012). For instance, children may have difficulties forming friendships because of school absenteeism or the different challenges they experience as a result of living with their chronic illness. Moreover, children may feel they are "different" or do not fit in with their peers. This feeling may initiate with the child, because he or she feels different due to having an illness. Although children face psychosocial difficulties and difficulties getting along with peers, many may get along well with peers and form strong friendships.

In addition to physical challenges, pediatric chronic illness can impact social and emotional development and health. Compared to their healthy counterparts, children living with a chronic illness may be more likely to present with mental health problems, including emotional disorders, behavioral issues and school-related adjustment problems and drop out (Blackman et al. 2011; Compas et al. 2012). Children with chronic illnesses may experience externalizing problems, but may also be more likely to experience internalizing problems, such as anxiety (Blackman et al. 2011; Ferro and Boyle 2015; Pinquart and Shen 2011). Moreover, they may be coping with trauma in the aftermath of repeated hospitalization and related invasive medical procedures. Despite these challenges, many children and adolescents function well, and providing them with strategies to promote their coping, such as with anxiety, can improve quality of life for children and adolescents with chronic illnesses.

COPING WITH ANXIETY AND WORRY

Children and adolescents with chronic illnesses may experience anxiety and worry related to medical procedures, the course of their illness, and hospitalizations (Pinquart and Shen 2011). Kendall, Settipani, and Cummings (2012) noted that cognitive-behavioral coping strategies (new ways to think and act) can be very useful in helping children reduce anxiety. In our team's work (e.g., Nabors et al. 2019a), we have found that children and teenagers report using coping strategies, and often benefit from distraction and calming strategies when they face medical procedures and repeated hospitalizations. We have used cognitive-behavioral anxiety management strategies, including breathing, muscle relaxation, positive imagery and positive self-talk to help young children manage anxiety related to their illnesses. As we have worked with children, it has been clear that social support is valuable, both that of family and friends. Children often rely on siblings for family and peer support, either when siblings are with them at a nearby Ronald McDonald House (housing for families with a child with a chronic illness) or through keeping in touch electronically, such as via FaceTime or Skype (Nabors et al. 2019a). Similar to Dahlquist et al. (2002), we have found that distraction is a highly valued strategy for coping with painful medical procedures.

We have found that children are fairly resilient and use family support to help build their resilience (e.g., Nabors et al. 2019b). Many have developed their own coping strategies, and these strategies are often maximized if they have worked with a pediatric psychologist (Nabors et al. 2019a). For example, young children can use favorite stuffed animals and electronics for distraction during procedures or for comfort when they are bored during hospitalization. Children and older youth also use games, often on the iPad or iPhone as distraction, and thus should be allowed access to these accessories. When we asked children about what type of self-statements they needed to speak encouragingly to themselves, many often reported needing a "can do" or "I can do it" mantra so that they were positive when facing painful procedures or upset about being in the hospital. Others used music to calm themselves and often had special songs that built their confidence and sense of being calm and able to handle procedures and hospitalization (Nabors et al. 2019b). We also believe that parents can be coaches, working to praise positive coping efforts by their children. It can be easy for parents to accidentally reinforce upset and panic during procedures, and with coaching from health professionals, parents can be assets for children. This coaching role can benefit parents as they feel useful and have a role on their child's medical team.

RESILIENCE

Children with chronic illnesses and their families may, for the most part, be marked by resilience and positive functioning. Alvord and Grados (2005) defined resilience as the skills and attributes that allow persons to deal with difficulties or life stressors. Positive activities, such as positive self-talk and coping, which are critical to positive psychology, are related to positive mental health, which may promote resilience (Hamall et al., 2014). It is critical to consider family resilience, as child and adolescent functioning are inextricably intertwined with that of the family (e.g., Masten 2018). Masten's definition of resilience applies to the family, as a system. Masten (2018) stated that,

> ...resilience can be defined as follows: The capacity of a system to adapt successfully to significant challenges that threaten the function, viability, or development of the system. Thus, adapting in the face of stress is part of resilient system functioning (p. 16).

Froma Walsh (2003) discussed the importance of building family resilience by improving positive outlook and expressing emotions, which would, in turn, decrease stress for all individuals within a family. Similarly, developing strong social supports which contribute to positive feelings, such as building a strong network of family friends, can be resilience-building. Having a strong circle of support persons as a buffer in times of stress can be affirming and resilience-building for the child and his or her family members (Walsh 2002, 2003). Walsh (2002) proposed that, "...in family organization, resilience can be fostered through flexible structure, shared leadership, mutual support, and team work in facing challenges" (p. 132). Thus, a family that pulled together as a team, and found a new balance to deal with stress, was hardy, and resilient in its functioning.

More research on family resilience is needed, however, as results of studies assessing family functioning are mixed. For instance, researchers have proposed that families are marked by positive functioning and resilience (Chen, Brody, and Miller 2017; Mullins et al. 2015). Conversely, others have found that family members experience mental health problems and family members are at increased risk for dysfunction when a family member has an illness (e.g., Ferro and Boyle 2015). In fact, Zhang et al. (2015) suggested that hospitalization of a child may results in significant distress and poor adjustment for families.

Being hardy may be another factor that improves positive functioning when a family system faces a stressor, such as having a family member with a chronic illness. Families with high levels of hardiness are resilient, in that they can rely on one another, accept help from others, and learn new ways of coping when experiencing stressful situations (Walsh, 1998, 2002). Hardiness can occur at the individual and family levels. Olsen et al. (1999) defined hardiness as describing, "...people who remain healthy even while experiencing high amounts of life stress. It is thought to contain three components: control, commitment and challenge" (p. 277). People who are hardy believe that they can do things to affect stress, are committed to acting in positive ways, and perform resilient and positive actions in the face of challenges. Family hardiness refers to the cohesive unit and its strengths in this manner,

> "Family hardiness refers to the internal strengths and durability of the family unit and is characterized by a sense of control over the outcomes of life events and hardships, a view of change as advantageous and growth producing, and an active rather than passive orientation in adjusting to and managing stressful situations" (p. 278, Olsen et al. 1999).

McCubbin et al. (2002) studied families with a child who was battling cancer. They found that these families were hardy, with resilience at their core, in trying to adjust to the child's illness. Families who tended to cope well displayed factors including: an absence of marital problems, high marital relationship quality, and good coping of other family members (McCubbin et al. 2002).

Positive psychology may have a role in shaping resilience in children and families. An overarching goal of this field is to improve individual's feelings of satisfaction with life and the past, well-being, optimism, and happiness (Seligman and Csikszentmihalyi 2000). In regards to the individual level, this field focuses on a person's positive traits, such as resilience, and on building positive emotional responses in order to cope with stressors (Seligman and Csikszentmihalyi 2000). Interventions that utilize positive psychology may decrease negative emotional problems and increase resilience among individuals, providing more positive meaning in life. It is important to use strategies from positive psychology, such as positive thinking and self-talk, to build the resilience of youth with chronic illnesses. This will promote positive emotional and behavioral functioning that will enhance their well-being (Hamall et al. 2014). One way to do this is to boost resilience, by increasing the child's feelings of hope and optimism as well as his or her abilities to engage in positive thinking (Seligman 1995). In addition, teaching problem-solving skills, relaxation, and positive self-talk may be other ways to boost resilience in children facing chronic illnesses (Nabors et al.2019a).

PARENTS AND SIBLINGS: THEIR ROLE AS HELPERS AND THEIR NEEDS FOR SUPPORT

Parents also can be marked by resilience. They may cope well when they feel they are maintaining their role as nurturers. As such, it can be beneficial for both the child and his or her parent, when the parent has a role in supporting the child during medical procedures and explaining illness-related procedures to the child. Parents may be instrumental in their role as cheerleaders and coaches – encouraging children in the family and striving to help them maintain a normal life and "just be children." We believe parents can benefit from education on the cognitive-behavioral strategies presented in this chapter. If parents learn these strategies and can assist their children in using them, they can support their children during painful and stressful procedures, when the therapist might not be present.

Parents also benefit from being supported by others. Parents may find support in extended family and friends, which is a source of comfort and support. Extended family may help the family maintain its routine when one parent and a child have to go to the hospital. Parents may need support from a therapist, especially in cases where the parent experiences trauma and stress related to their child's medical treatment. Parents may need support as they cope with financial stress, because they have to miss work or have medical expenses. Like their child, parents can experience "numbing" when it becomes overwhelming to watch their child face medical procedures and experience trauma. Parents may suppress their stress and trauma reactions, in order to support their child. Therapy can become a safe space for a parent to process grief and receive support while coping with a child's illness. Other parents may need to share feelings of distress with a close friend or family member as they become resolved to their child's illness and move through grief related to their child's illness and medical procedures he or she must face. Another area for discussion may be processing ways to support siblings should they experience jealousy or sadness as a parent's time can be monopolized by the many demands of the child's illness.

Siblings feel anxious about outcomes for their brother or sister with an illness or feel guilty because they are healthy, which may cause them stress and concomitantly to experience anxiety (Sharpe and Rossiter 2002). They may feel jealous of parental attention directed toward the child with an illness, especially when that child is away from home and undergoing medical procedures in a hospital (Williams et al. 2009). On the other hand, siblings can show considerable strength and resilience. For example, caring for a brother or sister may improve their understanding of the illness and increase their feelings of self-worth because they are part of the "care" team (Incledon et al. 2015; Sharpe and Rossiter 2002). Siblings may be a support for parents in their care-taking role as well. Siblings may take on parenting roles, caring for other younger siblings, to help parents, further strengthening their feelings of self-worth. Being a support person, such as by visiting the hospital or staying with the family at a Ronald McDonald House, can increase support for the child who is ill, and boost positive attitudes for siblings as well (Nabors, Liddle, et al., 2019). Connections and attachments improve resilience (Alvord and Grados 2005). We believe that parents and siblings being present and the family battling the illness as a team can strengthen the resilience of all family members through positive connection, shared purpose, and support.

THERAPIST'S ROLE

In the preceding sections of this chapter, we have highlighted the therapist's role in helping children cope with trauma by drawing from the literature related to the use of cognitive and behavioral techniques with children. These techniques are consistent with a positive coping framework, and therefore "fit" within our positive psychology framework. We would first like to highlight the use of relaxation and distraction as coping strategies which are presented in Table 1 (information is adapted from Nabors and Elkins 2017).

Table 1. Relaxation and Distraction Strategies

Relaxation	Distraction
Rock Sponge First, be a rock. Then be a sponge. You can relax and squeeze away the worry to reset your system. Relax by practicing making muscles tight like a rock and then relaxing like a sponge and taking deep breaths. The sponge squeezes out the worry. Now, it is your turn practice being the super relaxation sponge kid. Here is what you do… Sit in a chair or you can lay in your bed. Make your muscles tight, like a rock (when you do this, if a part of you hurts, do not make it like a rock! Just do the rock where it does not hurt). Then, make your muscles loose, like a sponge sinking in to your chair or bed. Take some deep breaths and close your eyes. Focus on Your Breathing Close your eyes. Breathe in nice and slow. Imagine your tummy is a beach ball and you are slowly filling it with air you breathe in. Hold the beach ball inside your belly until you count to five on your fingers. Now, slowly breathe out and imagine the beach ball slowly getting smaller. How many beach balls will you fill and make smaller to help shrink your worry? I will fill ( ) beach balls.	For distraction we discuss not focusing on what stresses us and taking a break from thinking about stressful things. Then, we talk about having fun and doing fun things as a form of distraction. After this, we list key distraction ideas, such as… Reading, playing on the iPad, playing a game, listening to music, working with Child Life specialists, and talking with friends and parents. We suggest using puzzles, watching movies, and playing videogames. Some children prefer to use a favorite toy or a special, soft blanket to distract themselves during medical procedures. We then have a child list three key distraction strategies he or she can use during painful or stressful medical procedures. A lot of children list parents and siblings – who give hugs and talk them through things – as critical under distraction strategies. This can be helpful. But, sometimes, we have the support of parents and friends stand alone in our menus or charts for the children. We write down all the ways parents and siblings support the child as its own category. This is because support of others who love us, in the form of kind words and hugs, is a powerful strategy.

Table 2. Imagery and Positive Self-Talk Strategies

Imagery: Imagine Your Happy Place	Positive Self-Talk and Positive Psych-up Phrases
Imagining a happy place can help you to take a break from your worries. Trudy's favorite spot is the beach. She thinks about the beach, ocean, and warm sun when she wants a vacation from her worries. Trudy likes to make sand castles and relax at the beach. She pretends the warm sun makes her worries get small. She sees a boat in the water. She hears the waves as they hit the sand. Can you see the beach? Can you hear the water? Now, is your worry smaller? Take a vacation from your worry...practice going to your favorite place in your imagination. What is your favorite place? What is it like? What happens there? What does it sound like? Is it warm or cold? What do you see? What are you doing? What happens next?	It is good to use positive talk against the worries. Positive talk mean saying to yourself, "I can deal with this needle stick, because I have had them before and it turned out OK." Or "I can deal with being in the hospital. I can help the doctors and nurses and talk to my family if I need to cheer up." Say positive things inside your head, like, "I can deal with this." "It will be OK, and I have lots of family and friends who care about me." "I can do it. I am special." If you catch the voice inside your head saying mean worry things over and over, that worry is growing. It is time to push pause. Then, you can stop the worries by using positive words. We have children develop their own positive coping words in thought bubbles above a picture of a "thinking emoji." We practice positive coping statements with the children and their parents. Teaching the child to praise him or herself for using positive phrases has been an important part of our practice.

We believe that both types of strategies should be selected in cooperation with the child and his or her parents (ideas are from a coping manual, entitled, *"Coping Positively with My Worries Manual for Kids,"* developed by Nabors and Elkins 2017).

In addition, we use positive self-talk and positive imagery, which we design based on what works for the child. Examples of how we introduce the notion of positive self-talk and positive imagery, which often works as a distraction tool, are presented in Table 2 (information is adapted from Nabors and Elkins 2017).

In terms of imagery, we discuss finding a child's happy place, which could be going to an amusement park. We ask the child to visit this place in his or her mind, and experience it with all his or her senses, such as hearing the sounds, seeing all the details, etc. (see Table 2). Sometimes, especially if children are younger, we work with them to select a superhero to help them fight pain or worry with positive images and deeds. For positive self-talk, we help the child select personal mantras that the child can repeat during times of stress, such as "I can do it! Charge! I can beat my pain." We try to assemble all of the children's strategies on a coping menu or notecard that they can take with them (Nabors and Elkins 2017; Nabors et al. 2019a). Teaching and reminding children to use self-praise and parents to praise the child for positive coping has been a critical component of our work. We do a lot of supportive listening too, as the children have stories that they need to share and grief that needs to be processed. Thus, therapists and health professionals may be able to adapt techniques from the trauma informed care literature to help children, and other family members, as they cope with stress and grief related to having a chronic illness.

IDEAS FOR THERAPISTS FROM TRAUMA INFORMED CARE

Aspects of the trauma coping literature can be applied to assisting children with chronic illnesses. Therapists need to become knowledgeable about helping children cope with anxiety and stress, anger related to having an illness, feelings of powerlessness over the illness and its waxing and waning course, and feeling a lack of control over one's body. In some cases, children with chronic illnesses experience depression related to low self-esteem, repeated hospitalizations, and feeling a sense of hopelessness. The therapy session may be a place where children can express their frustrations and feel a sense of safety, allowing them to express feelings related to the trauma of repeated hospitalizations. This safe space, in turn, allows for catharsis, which can begin a healing process. Improving the child's support at home and increasing friendships and involvement in positive activities can be supportive as well, helping to lift children's spirits. It is beneficial to become well versed in activities that build a child's feelings of optimism and self-esteem (e.g., Seligman 1995). We have found that helping the child identify personal strengths and hobbies can boost his or her self-esteem. Some children with chronic illnesses may feel they are different from others their age, and for some, teasing or stigma related to their illness (e.g., such as stigma for children with gastrointestinal problems) may decrease their motivation to establish friendships with peers. In these cases, the therapist may be able to promote resilience by teaching the child friendship skills, helping him or her join support groups, or explain the illness to peers at school.

Trauma may be related to feelings of depression. In order to address trauma reactions, the therapist can help the child understand the trauma and tell his or her "story." While listening, the therapist can assist the child in coping with his or her illness and help the child learn about ways to consolidate grief related to his or her illness into the story of his or her life. The therapist can aid the child in comprehending that intrusive, negative thoughts about medical procedures may be a form of flashbacks. These flashbacks can be a way of working through upsetting feelings. In other instances, some children may be hyper-aroused in medical situations, if past negative experiences have occurred. Anxiety management techniques, especially relaxation techniques, may be important tools if the child must undergo further medical procedures. On the other hand, a child may experience emotional numbing, seeming to have a very flat affect, if he or she is overwhelmed by trauma. The therapist may need to help the child recall stressful situations, in order for the child to become able to express emotions, and therefore become more open to experiencing emotions or "feeling" different types of emotions. In these instances, the therapy session may become a "safe space," where children can fully express themselves without worrying about upsetting their parents. Thus, therapists working with children with chronic illness may benefit from becoming well-versed in techniques and interventions for "trauma informed care." One possible resource in this area is the Child Welfare Information Gateway (www.childwelfare.gov/pubs/trauma) and another source of information is the Center for Traumatic Stress in Children at Pittsburgh (www.pittsburghchildtrauma.com). Cohen and colleagues have written many beneficial articles on trauma informed care using cognitive and behavioral techniques (e.g., Cohen, Berliner, and Mannarino 2000; Cohen et al. 2000).

The Complex Trauma Workgroup (CTWG) of the National Child Traumatic Stress Network identified components of interventions for trauma (Cook et al. 2005). Emotional dysregulation, including significant anxiety, may be a common experience for youth who have experienced trauma. Other symptoms associated with trauma are behavioral dysregulation, difficulty attaching securely with others, and poor self-concept. Treatment of complex trauma involves teaching children how to cope with anxiety, feel safe, regulate emotions and behaviors, and reducing feelings of worry that cause hypervigilance and difficulties with cognitive processing. It involves helping the child understand (making meaning in his or her own words and with his or her own ideas) his or her traumatic experiences. Therapists also help children improve attachments to (or relational engagement with) others and improve feelings of self-worth. Interventions for improving positive affect and regulating anxiety and emotions, such as using mindfulness and relaxation, may be especially helpful for youth who have had traumatic experiences (Cook et al. 2005). In a similar fashion, family members can experience "vicarious" trauma and need referral to a counselor to help them cope and find hope for the future. Newcomb, Moore, and Matto (2018) describe key processes for supporting family members and patients to improve hope and positive functioning in the community. They provide critical recommendations for case management and improving connections with others with their HOPE for Families Model, which stresses having family members work together as they cope with the illness of a family member.

If the child is experiencing depression, the therapist needs to ensure that the child is not experiencing suicidal ideation and is sleeping and eating within normal limits. If suicidal ideation or depression is severe, referral for a medication evaluation by a psychiatrist may be indicated. In other instances, hospitalization may be warranted. Moreover, if the child is not eating or sleeping according to normal patterns, the therapist needs to encourage the child resume a sleep routine and begin the eat nutritiously, especially if the child is taking many medications related to his or her illness. Additionally, with any referral to a psychiatrist for evaluation, it may be important to alert the medical team and seek their advice, if the child is on a complex medication regimen due to his or her illness.

STRATEGIES FOR FAMILIES

There are many strategies that may assist families as they cope with a child's chronic illness. We would like to mention a few of our ideas. One is to find a "helping role" for all family members so that they all can feel they are pulling as a team to help in facing the stressor, which is the chronic illness. This can include finding a role for siblings as friends and positive cheerleaders. They can provide support through FaceTime and telephone calls. Parents can learn cognitive-behavioral techniques, such as the anxiety management techniques we mentioned in this chapter, so that they can become coaches at the hospital and when the child needs to relax and manage anxiety. If necessary referral to therapy can be helpful, especially in times of stress for the family. Another idea to promote resilience is to help members of the family process grief related to the loss of normal lives they and the child with an illness must face. Most families will come to terms with a stressor and make meaning of it, weaving this new normal into the fabric of their family life. We also believe that being with other families, either through attending support groups, having a mentor, or staying at a local Ronald McDonald House (with other families with a child with an illness) can be a support for families and children. For instance, families have other families for support at local Ronald McDonald Houses, and parents may find the social support they need there, as might siblings, who often need support too. It is nice to know that one is not alone, and that others are coping with similar stressors and finding their way toward resilience and meaning as they cope. Similarly, summer camps for children who face the same chronic illnesses may be a support for the child who is battling the illness. Other types of social support from family and friends may help the family find balance, as all members of the family move toward a new normal (e.g., finding a new way of functioning) in coping with each different phase, and the waxing and waning symptoms, of most chronic illnesses.

CONCLUSION

This chapter has summarized ideas for helping children cope with anxiety, which will promote their resilience as they deal with procedures and hospitalizations related to their chronic illnesses. Cognitive-behavioral techniques have a solid evidence base, in terms of their effectiveness in helping children cope with anxiety (e.g., Kendall et al. 2012). The cognitive-behavioral strategies, in addition to reducing anxiety, are linked to positive attitude. Positive thoughts and self-talk are a hallmark of positive psychology, and improving positive attitudes may improve positive functioning for individuals (Seligman and Csikszentmihalyi 2000). In his book on optimism for children, Seligman also posits that learning optimism can improve and maximize child functioning (Seligman 1995). We did note that for some children with chronic illnesses, especially those that have faced many medical procedures and hospitalizations, trauma may result. If children or family members (who may experience vicarious trauma) have experienced significant trauma referral for therapy may be indicated. Therapists can draw from the evidence base developed for trauma informed care and provide therapeutic support to help children deal with feelings of trauma related to their medical condition (e.g., Cohen et al. 2000).

Moreover, we have discussed the concept of family resilience, and noted that families move toward resilience and thus might be characterized as "resilient" or bouncing back in a positive way as they cope with a child's chronic illness. Resilience is a balancing act, as the family or system develops new strategies to cope with a stressor and make meaning of it, so that the family members' lives can move forward to be the best they can be (Masten 2018; Walsh 2003). Those families that function positively fairly quickly and who bounce back quickly in the face of stress may be characterized as "hardy" (e.g., Olsen et al. 1999). Factors related to hardiness may be having a positive attitude, being able to express emotions (both positive and negative), having social support, and being able to communicate about problems within the family. Future research will be needed to better understand factors that strengthen the hardiness to resilience link. When we gain improved understanding of these factors and how to promote them, there may be further gains in family resilience and we may be able to develop interventions based on a positive psychology framework to continue to strengthen family functioning.

REFERENCES

Algozzine, Bob and Jim Ysseldyke 2006. *Teaching students with medical, physical, and multiple disabilities: A practical guide for every teacher.* Thousand Oaks, CA: Corwin.

Alvord, Mary Karapetuab, and Judy J. Grados. 2005. "Enhancing Resilience in Children: A Proactive Approach." *Professional Psychology: Research and Practice* 36:238-245. doi: 10.1037/0735-7028.36.3.238.

Bethell, Christina, D., Michael D. Kogan, Bonnie B. Strickland, Edward L. Schor, Julie Robertson and Paul W. Newacheck. 2011. "A National and State Profile of Leading Health Problems with Healthcare Quality for U.S. Children: Key Insurance Disparities and Across-State Variations." *Academic Pediatrics* 11(3 Supp):S22-S33. doi: 10.1016/j.acap.2010.08.011.

Blackman, James A., Matthew J. Gurka, Kelly K. Gurka and Oliver M. Norman. 2011. "Emotional, Developmental and Behavioural Co-morbidities of Children with Chronic Health Conditions." *Journal of Paediatrics and Child Health* 47:742-747. doi:10.1111/j.1440-1754.2011.02044.x.

Chen, Edith, Gene H. Brody and Gregory E. Miller. 2017. "Childhood Close Family Relationships and Health." *American Psychologist* 72:555-566. doi: 10.1037/amp0000067.

Churchill, Shervin S., Nanci L. Villareale, Teresa A. Monaghan, Virginia L. Sharp and Gail M. Kieckhefer. 2010. "Parents of Children with Special Health Care Needs Who Have Better Coping Skills have Fewer Depressive Symptoms." *Maternal and Child Health Journal* 14:47-57. doi: 10.1007/s10995-008-0435-0.

Cohen, Judith A., Lucy Berliner and Anthony P. Mannarino. 2000. "Treatment of Traumatized Children: A Review and Synthesis. *Trauma, Violence, and Abuse* 1:29-46. doi: 10.1177/15248380000 01001003.

Cohen, Judith A., Anthony P. Mannarino, Lucy Berliner and Esther Deblinger. 2000. "Trauma-Focused Cognitive Behavioral Therapy: An Empirical Update." *Journal of Interpersonal Violence* 15:1203-1223. https://pdfs.semanticscholar.org/7302/e6a76089a25fd0c1714a0388565 a5e0eeb79.pdf.

Compas, Bruce E., Sarah S. Jaser, Madeleine J. Dunn and Erin M. Rodriguez. 2012. "Coping with Chronic Illness in Childhood and Adolescence." *Annual Review of Clinical Psychology* 8:455–480. doi: 10.1146/annurev-clinpsy-032511-143108.

Cook, Alexandra, Joseph Spinazzola, Julian Ford, Cheryl Lanktree, Margaret Blaustein, Marylene Cloitre, M.,…and Bessel van der Kolk. 2005. "Complex Trauma in Children and Adolescents." *Psychiatric Annals* 35:390-398. doi: 10.3928/00485713-20050501-05.

Dahlquist, Lynnda M., Suzanne M. Busby, Keith J. Slifer, Cindy L. Tucker, Stephanie Eischen, Lisa Hilley and Wendy Sulc. 2002. "Distraction for Children of Different Ages Who Undergo Repeated Needle Sticks." *Journal of Pediatric Oncology Nursing* 19:22-34. doi: 10.1053/jpon.2002.30009.

Mark A. Ferro and Michael H. Boyle. 2015. "The Impact of Chronic Physical Illness, Maternal Depressive Symptoms, Family Functioning, and Self-Esteem on Symptoms of Anxiety and Depression in

Children." *Journal of Abnormal Child Psychology* 43:177-187. doi: 10.1007/s10802-014-9893-6.

Gannoni, Anne, F. and Rosalyn H. Shute. 2010. "Parental and Child Perspectives on Adaptation to Childhood Chronic Illness: A Qualitative Study." *Clinical Child Psychology and Psychiatry* 15:39–53. doi: 10.1177/1359104509338432.

Hamall, Katrina, M, Todd R. Heard, Kerry J. Inder, Katherine M. McGill and Frances Kay-Lambkin. 2014. "The Child Illness and Resilience Program (CHiRP): A Study Protocol of a Stepped Care Intervention to Improve the Resilience and Wellbeing of Families Living with Childhood Chronic Illness." *BMC Psychology* 2:5 (10 pages). doi: 10.1186/2050-7283-2-5.

Incledon, Emily, Lauren Williams, Trevor Hazell, Todd R. Heard, Alexandra Flowers and Harriet Hiscock. 2015. "A Review of Factors Associated with Mental Health in Siblings of Children with Chronic Illnesses." *Journal of Child Health Care* 19:182-194. doi: 10.1177/1367493513503584.

Kendall, Phillip C., Cara A. Settipani and Colleen M. Cummings. 2012. "No Need to Worry: The Promising Future of Child Anxiety Research." *Journal of Clinical Child and Adolescent Psychology* 41:103-115. doi: 10.1080/15374416.2012.632352.

Martire, Lynn M. and Vicki S. Helgeson. 2017. "Close Relationships and the Management of Chronic Illness: Associations and Interventions." *American Psychologist* 72:601-612. doi: 10.1037/amp0000066.

Masten, Anne S. 2018. "Resilience Theory and Research on Children and Families: Past, Present, and Promise." *Journal of Family Theory and Review* 10:12-31. doi: 10.1111/jftr.12255.

McCubbin, Marilyn, Karla Balling, Peggy Possin, Sharon Frierdich and Barbara Bryne. 2002. "Family Resiliency in Childhood Cancer." *Family Relations* 51:103-111. doi: 10.1111/j.1741-3729.2002.00103.x.

Mullins. Larry L., Elizabeth S. Molzon, Kristina I. Suorsa, Alayna P. Tackett, Ahna L. H. Pai and John M. Chaney. 2015. "Models of Resilience: Developing Psychosocial Interventions for Parents of

Children with Chronic Health Conditions." *Family Relations* 64:176-189. doi: 10.1111/fare.12104.

Nabors, Laura, and JaLisa Elkins. 2017. *Coping Positively with My Worries Manual for Kids.* University of Cincinnati, Cincinnati, Ohio, Author.

Nabors, Laura, Cathleen Odar Stough, Angela Combs and JaLisa Elkins. 2019(a). Implementing the Coping Positively with My Worries Manual: A Pilot Study. *Journal of Child and Family Studies* Published early online, 10 pp. Accessed July 18, 2019. https://link. springer.com/article/10.1007%2Fs10826-019-01451-3.

Nabors, Laura, Melissa Liddle, Myia Lang Graves, Allison Kamphaus and JaLisa Elkins. 2019(b). A Family Affair: Supporting Children with Chronic Illnesses. *Child: Care, Health and Development* 45:227–233. doi: 10.1111/cch.12635.

Newcomb, Anna, L Gordon Moore and Holly C. Matto. 2018. Family Centered Caregiving from Hospital to Home: Coping with Trauma and Building Capacity within the HOPE for Families Model. *Patient Experience Journal*, 5, Article 10: pp. 66-75. Accessed July 18, 2019. http://pxjournal.org/journal/vol5/iss1/10.

Ollendick, Thomas, H. and Carolyn S. Schroeder. 2003. *Encyclopedia of clinical child and pediatric psychology.* New York: Kluwer Academic/Plenum Publishers.

Olsen, Susanne F., Elaine S. Marshall, Barbara L. Mandleco, Keith W. Allred, Tina T. Dyches, and Nancy Sansom. 1999. Support, Communication, and Hardiness in Families with Children with Disabilities. *Journal of Family Nursing* 5:275-291. doi: 10.1177/ 107484079900500303.

Pinquart, Martin. 2013. Self-esteem of Children and Adolescents with Chronic Illness: A Meta-Analysis. *Child: Care, Health and Development* 39:153-61. doi: 10.1111/j.1365-2214.2012.01397.

Pinquart, Martin and Yuhui Shen. 2011. Anxiety in Children and Adolescents with Chronic Physical Illnesses: A Meta-Analysis. *Acta Paediatrica* 100:1069-1076. doi: 10.1111/j.1651-2227.2011.02223.x.

Seligman, Martin E. 1995. *The Optimistic Child: A Revolutionary Program that Safeguards Children Against Depression & Builds Lifelong Resilience*. Boston: Houghton Mifflin.

Seligman, Martin E. and Mihaly Csikszentmihalyi, M. (2000). Positive Psychology: An introduction. *American Psychologist* 55:5-14. doi.org/10.1037/0003-066X.55.1.5.

Sharpe, Donald, and Lucille Rossiter. 2002. Siblings of Children with a Chronic Illness: A Meta-Analysis. *Journal of Pediatric Psychology* 27:699-710. doi: 10.1093/jpepsy/27.8.699.

Trowbridge, Kelly and Lisa Mische-Lawson. 2014. Families with Children with Medical Complexity and Self-management of Care: A Systematic Review of the Literature. *Social Work in Health Care* 53:640-658. doi: 10.1080/00981389.2014.916776.

Walsh, Froma. 1998. *Strengthening Family Resilience*. New York: Guilford Press.

Walsh, Froma. 2002. A Family Resilience Framework: Innovative Practice Applications. *Family Relations* 51: 130-137. doi.org/10.1111/j.1741-3729.2002.00130.x.

Walsh, Froma. 2003. Family Resilience: A Framework for Clinical Practice. *Family Process* 42:1-18. *doi: 10.1111/j.1545-5300.2003.00001.x.*

Williams, Phoebe Dauz, E. Lavonne Ridder, Robyn K. Setter, Adrienne Liebergen, Heather Curry, Ubolrat Piamjariyakul, and Arthur R. Williams. 2009. Pediatric Chronic Illness (Cancer, Cystic Ribrosis) Effects on Well Siblings: Parents' Voices. *Issues in Comprehensive Pediatric Nursing* 32:94-113. doi: 10.1080/01460860902740990.

Zhang, Y., Wei, M., Shen, N., & Zhang, Y. (2015). Identifying Factors Related to Family Management During the Coping Process of Families with Childhood Chronic Conditions: A Multi-Site Study. *Journal of Pediatric Nursing* 30:160-173. doi: 10.1016/j.pedn.2014.10.002.

In: Coping with Chronic Illness   ISBN: 978-1-53616-775-7
Editor: Meghan Mendoza   © 2020 Nova Science Publishers, Inc.

Chapter 4

QUALITY OF LIFE IN WOMEN WITH BREAST CANCER

Inês Pereira[1], Marta Pereira[1], Ângela Leite[2] and M. Graça Pereira[3]

[1] School of Psychology, University of Minho, Braga, Portugal
[2] Psychology Research Center (CIPsi), University of Minho, Braga, Portugal
[3] School of Psychology, University of Minho, Braga, Portugal; Psychology Research Center (CIPsi), Braga, Portugal

ABSTRACT

Breast cancer is the most common malignant tumor in women. Chemotherapy is an adjuvant systemic therapy often used as a treatment for breast cancer with a significant impact on reducing the risk of relapse and overall mortality but with adverse effects on the emotional and functional domains of the patient's life. Women present greater psychological morbidity, higher levels of stress revealed by deregulated cortisol patterns, which are associated with a worse prognosis and tumor growth, less efficient coping strategies and more negative illness perceptions. This chapter reviews and analyzes the relationship among sociodemographic and clinical variables, psychological morbidity, self-efficacy for coping, illness perceptions and quality of life taking into consideration disease stage. The results showed that coping was positively associated with quality of life. Disease stage, treatment side effects, anxiety, depression, illness perceptions and cortisol awakening response (CAR) correlated negatively with QoL. The results suggest that these variables should be considered from the beginning of chemotherapy in interventions and individualized programs adapted to the psychological needs of these patients.

Keywords: Quality of life, chemotherapy, cortisol, self-efficacy for coping, illness perceptions, psychological morbidity

INTRODUCTION

Breast cancer (BC) occurs when breast cells grow in an uncontrolled way, originating tumors that may invade adjacent tissues, or metastasize to other more distant tissues in the human body. According to Bray et al. (2018), this is the most common type of cancer in women worldwide, corresponding to 2,088849 new cases in 2018, accounting for 11.6% of all tumors detected, being the most frequent cause of death in 11 regions of the world such as Ferlay et al. (2018) stated. It is estimated that, in 2019, in the United States, there are 268,600 new cases of BC in women and 41,760 deaths. There is no single cause known for this disease, but it is known that there are factors that contribute for its development, such as family history, age, and personal history, among others (Colditz, Kaphingst, Hankinson, & Rosner, 2012; Kotsopoulos et al., 2010; National Cancer Institute, 2019).

In the initial stages of BC, usually, there is no symptoms or pain and for this reason, any observable physical change is important (National Cancer Institute, 2019). BC diagnosis is established through clinical examination: palpation, biopsy and imaging tests. Subsequently, and depending on the results, the most appropriate treatment is defined and may include surgery, chemotherapy, radiotherapy, hormone therapy and/or targeted therapies (National Cancer Institute, 2019). The disease stage is defined according to the TNM system (Tumor, Node, and Metastasis), that range from zero to four and is essential to assist in clinical decision making regarding the therapy to be adopted for the patient (Gannon, Cotter, & Quinn, 2013; Singletary et al., 2003). Noninvasive cancers are classified as stage 0, meaning that adjacent/contiguous areas are not affected. The stages from I to III are invasive; the cancer may have spread to nearby. Finally, in stage IV, BC is spread to distant parts of the body (Shead et al., 2012; Shead, Hanisch, Vidic, Corrigan, & Clarke, 2018).

One of the most common treatments for BC is surgery. In the surgical process, the tumor can be removed keeping what is left of the breast (conservative breast surgery); mammary tissue can be totally removed (mastectomy); or the breast is removed as well as most or all axillary lymph nodes (modified radical mastectomy). Another type of treatment is chemotherapy and requires the use of drugs to eliminate the cancer cells. However, it has undesirable side effects such as patients becoming more likely to suffer from infections, bruising or bleeding easily, feeling weak and tired, suffering from hair loss and/or manifesting loss of appetite, nausea/ vomiting, diarrhea and mouth sores (National Cancer Institute, 2019). In the study of Bushatsky et al. (2017), patients reported that the side effects of systemic treatment were what most interfered in their daily lives. Kamińska et al. (2015) stated that, of all symptoms reported by patients undergoing mastectomy, the most difficult to deal with were nausea and vomiting. For Villar et al. (2017), the most disturbing symptoms were insomnia, fatigue and concern about hair loss. Although chemotherapy has a very important action in this process, such as tumor reduction, it is extremely relevant to consider its impact on the patient's physical, psychological and social functioning regarding quality of life (QoL).

The chemotherapeutic treatment impacts QoL, mostly the emotional and functional domains (Bushatsky et al., 2017). Only a few dimensions of QoL improve (emotional function and future perspectives), while physical function, role, body image, financial concerns and symptomatology worsen (Kamińska et al., 2015; Villar et al., 2017; Wöckel et al., 2017). In a study of Sha (2018), the overall health status of QoL was positively related to the emotional functioning and negatively with breast symptoms, arm symptoms and hair loss that were significant predictors of fatigue, pain, body image. However, there are some studies reporting that QoL is not affected and is therefore perceived by the patients as satisfactory (Costa et al., 2017; Lostaunau, Torrejón, & Cassaretto, 2017; Sousa, Guerra, & Lencastre, 2015). Between surgery and the beginning of adjuvant treatment, BC patients, when compared to a control group, had lower scores in overall health and functional role, emotional and social domains, and higher scores of fatigue, pain and loss of appetite (Debess, Riis, Pedersen, & Ewertz, 2009). Women who underwent radical surgery (lumpectomy) had worse QoL (physical function, pain, functional scale, symptoms and body image), while those who underwent conservative surgery had relatively good QoL (Boing et al., 2017; Kamińska et al., 2015). Tiezzi et al. (2017) found that chemotherapy treatment for breast cancer lowers QoL in the physical functioning and the role-physical domains of the SF-36 compared with women treated without chemotherapy. Besides, Kamińska et al. (2015) found that chemotherapy by itself could impair certain physical functions and had a negative impact on QoL. Kaptein et al. (2013) reported that, in a sample of Japanese and Dutch women, overall health, physical functioning, functional performance and emotional function were affected. In fact, women felt more fatigue, nausea, insomnia, loss of appetite, diarrhea and constipation one week after the first chemotherapy cycle and, eight weeks later, the results remained. A study by Costa et al. (2017) found that cancer patients suffered loss of functional capability (i.e., degree of dependence and disability) in a single cycle of chemotherapy, which was also associated with a reduction in QoL (Tang et al., 2017).

Patients with BC under 50 years old, when compared with the normative population, showed lower emotional functioning and higher levels of anxiety and depressive symptoms after diagnosis (Høyer et al., 2011). In addition, patients also presented significantly higher levels of anxiety and depression after surgery; it was higher in women undergoing mastectomy who had already completed chemotherapy treatment (Debess et al., 2009; Kamińska et al., 2015). Mastectomized patients aged 35-44 years were more depressed and anxious than older women (aged 55 to 65 years) (Geyikci, Cakmak, Demirkol, & Uguz, 2018) with depression and anxiety being positively associated. In a sample of 112 women, more than one-third were anxious and about one-fourth showed depression, with no significant differences between the chemotherapy and the non-chemotherapy group (Tiezzi et al., 2017). A study by Bidstrup et al. (2015) revealed that BC patients who received chemotherapy reported high levels of distress and depression and, of 323 newly diagnosed women, 8% had chronic and severe distress. In the study, being younger, having no partner, having less education and receiving chemotherapy were associated with more severe distress (Bidstrup et al., 2015) and younger age was associated with anxiety and depression. There was also an association between the extent of surgery and the degree of psychological distress, since the latter increased proportionally with the first (Schubart et al., 2014). However, in a study carried out in Portugal, participants did not present depressive symptomatology, but the anxious symptoms were more evident (Sousa et al., 2015).

> Higher rates of depression, anxiety, and moderate or severe distress were associated with worse QoL (Head et al., 2012; Patoo, Moradi, & Payandeh, 2014; Rebholz et al., 2016; Sousa et al., 2015; Tang et al., 2017). In one of these studies, we found a significant negative association between depression and anxiety and domains of QoL, including physical, role, emotional, functional, cognitive and social and a positive association with symptoms of pain and fatigue (Patoo et al., 2014).

Some studies have found that negative psychological results resulting from BC cause a disruption in cortisol rhythms (Bower et al., 2005; Giese-Davis et al., 2006). Cortisol is a glucocorticoid involved in stress response and is described as one of the main stress hormones, which is involved in energy metabolism and circadian rhythm regulation (Barsevick, Frost, Zwinderman, Hall, & Halyard, 2010). In a study by Zeitzer et al. (2016), altered nadir cortisol levels were associated with cancer progression. In fact, BC patients on chemotherapeutic treatment have significantly higher levels of cortisol when compared with healthy individuals, suggesting that they experience higher levels of stress (Abercrombie et al., 2004; Loo et al., 2013). Dysregulated cortisol patterns were associated with poorer QoL (Armer et al., 2018), increasing the expression of side effects by suppressing the immune system (Sephton et al., 2000), which, in turn, was associated with poorer QoL (Sha, 2018). Thus, it is important to understand the cortisol moderating role in the relationship between side effects and QoL.

According to García et al. (2016), coping strategies have a great influence on cortisol levels and explained 55% of its variation. Coping also correlates with QoL. In fact, negative coping predicts the subsequent QoL (Paek, Ip, Levine, & Avis, 2016). In a study by Farajzadegan, Khalili and Mokarian (2015), when coping skills were intervened, QoL improved considerably. To overcome the situations caused by the diagnosis of cancer, it is important for the patient to have effective coping strategies and adjustment skills. Rottmann, Dalton, Christensen, Frederiksen and Johansen (2010) found that the impact of self-efficacy for coping on the emotional well-being of BC patients was mediated by the patient's preferred coping strategies. Thus, patients with high self-efficacy tend to have a fighting spirit and fewer worries and hopelessness that later predicted a better emotional well-being. Shelby et al. (2014) reported that patients with high self-efficacy may be able to process information related to symptoms and find appropriate ways to control them, thereby improving well-being and QoL and also better able to correctly associate symptoms with their cause, leading to a reduction of anxiety. According to Chirico et al. (2017), patients who felt more capable to cope with cancer (high self-efficacy) reported better QoL, despite having the same level of distress than patients who felt less capable. Similarly, Badana et al. (2019) found a higher self-efficacy to be associated with a better QoL.

Illness perceptions in women with BC have also been associated with important outcomes in the course of the disease (Kaptein et al., 2015). Patients with BC are more likely to believe that their disease is related to uncontrollable factors, and not to behavioral ones (Kaptein et al., 2013; Ma, Yan, Wu, & Huang, 2018). Ma et al. (2018) noted that illness perceptions explained a significant proportion of the variance of the QoL. Another study with women with BC also found that perceiving the disease as more negative and threatening was associated with lower QoL (Ashley, Marti, Jones, Velikova, & Wright, 2015; Tang et al., 2017). According to Ashley et al. (2015), the dimensions of emotional representations and identity were also predictors of QoL. In addition, Kaptein et al. (2015) found that illness perceptions had a clear association with QoL and with having performed a mastectomy. In a sample of women who have undergone a mastectomy, negative illness perceptions were correlated with worse QoL (Fanakidou et al., 2018). Patients who underwent chemotherapy perceived the disease as more cyclical when compared to women who experienced other types of treatment (Castro, Lawrenz, Romeiro, Lima, & Haas, 2016). BC was perceived as having more negative consequences when women were married or lived with a partner and being older was associated with a more negative emotional representation, less perception of personal control and more consequences of BC (Castro et al., 2016).

Since the studies that address the relationships between cortisol, psychological variables and QoL are scarce, it is important to increase knowledge about how these variables contribute to QoL, in order to develop programs to reduce the negative psychological impact of BC. The inclusion of a psychophysiological stress indicator, such as cortisol, emphasizes the importance of this study since in addition to help identify psychological needs of women with BC, when cortisol is dysregulated, there are important physical consequences that need to be studied. Therefore, the present study fills a gap in the literature and by including patients in the initial stages of the disease receiving an adjuvant treatment, instead of survivors, also contributes for an understanding of patients' coping early on, that may help to design intervention programs that foster coping in this population over time.

In order to understand the impact and the relationship between certain variables and QoL, this study was based on the Livneh's Model of Psychosocial Adaptation to Chronic Illness (2001). This model considers the process of adaptation to a chronic disease as a dynamic process comprising three phases. In the first phase, antecedents include the triggering events (the cause of the disease and the contextual variables). In the second phase, called the adjustment process, the model includes the reactions and responses at the onset of illness (psychological morbidity and cortisol levels) and contextual variables that influence each other associated with the disease (stage and disease duration, number of cycles of chemotherapy, type of surgery, medication, and side effects of the disease), socio-demographic characteristics (age, marital status, educational attainment, employment status), environmental features and characteristics associated with psychological attributes and personality traits (illness perceptions and self-efficacy for coping). In the last phase, QoL is the main outcome variable of the chronic disease.

This study aims to analyze the relationship between sociodemographic and clinical variables, psychological morbidity, self-efficacy for coping, illness perceptions, cortisol and QoL. It is expected that coping, age and self-efficacy will be positively correlated with QoL and that the duration of the disease, type of surgery, side effects, psychological morbidity, cortisol, and illness perceptions will be negatively correlated with QoL.

METHODS

Participants

The sample consisted of 112 women diagnosed with BC from four central hospitals, in the North of Portugal. The inclusion criteria were: women diagnosed with BC at stage 1 or 2, receiving adjuvant chemotherapy treatment (the second cycle of chemotherapy) and scoring between 0-2 in degree of disability and dependence according to the Zubrod scale (Zubrod et al., 1960). All participants diagnosed with a psychosis or with cognitive deficit documented in the patient's chart were excluded.

Instruments

Sociodemographic and Clinical Questionnaire

This questionnaire includes questions regarding the sociodemographic and clinical data: age, marital status, literacy, current professional situation and duration of the disease.

Research and Treatment of Cancer Quality of Life Questionnaire

(EORTC QLQ-C30; Aaronson et al., 1993; Portuguese version of Pais-Ribeiro, Pinto, & Santos, 2008).

The EORTC QLQ-C30 evaluates the QoL in cancer patients through 30 items. The questionnaire consists of nine scales: five functional (physical, cognitive, emotional, role performance and social), one of global health, three of symptoms (fatigue, pain, nausea/vomiting) and some additional items related to symptoms frequently reported (loss of appetite, insomnia, dyspnea, constipation, diarrhea and financial difficulties). The answers are rated on a Likert scale (1 to 7 for overall health status and 1 to 4 for other items). All scales are converted to scores ranging from 0 to 100. Higher scores on global health and functional scales indicate better QoL and regarding the additional items, worse. In the original version, the Cronbach's alphas ranged between.52 and .89 and in the Portuguese version, from .57 to .88. In this study, only the full scale was used, with an alpha of .86.

Supplementary Questionnaire Breast Cancer Module

(EORTC QLQ-BR23; Sprangers et al., 1996; Portuguese version of EORTC).

The QLQ-BR23 questionnaire evaluates the effects of adjuvant treatments and is composed of 23 items. It measures four functional scales (body image, future perspectives, sexual function and sexual pleasure) and symptoms (affected breast and arm, concerns about hair loss and side effects of systemic treatments), with Likert type response (1 to 4). All scales were converted into scores ranging from 0 to 100. High scores indicate worse QoL on the symptom scale; in the remaining scales, high scores indicate a better QoL. Cronbach's alpha in the original version ranged from .46 to .94. In this study, only the dimension of the side effects of the systemic treatments was used, with an alpha of .60.

Illness Perception Questionnaire

(IPQ-Brief; Broadbent et al., 2006; Portuguese version of Figueiras et al., 2010)

The IPQ-Brief evaluates illness perceptions through nine items and includes three subscales: cognitive perceptions (consequences, duration, personal control, control through treatment and identity), emotional (worry and emotions) and understanding of the disease and causal representations. A high total score indicates more threatening illness perceptions. The answers are rated on a Likert scale from 0 to 10. Cronbach's alpha of full scale is not available. In this study, the alpha of the total scale was .75.

Cancer Behavior Inventory-Brief Version

(CBI-B; Heitzmann et al., 2011; Research version by Pereira & Pereira, 2015)

This instrument includes 12 items to evaluate the self-efficacy for coping of cancer patients answered on a Likert scale from 1 (not at all confident) to 9 (fully confident). Higher scores indicate greater self-efficacy in dealing with cancer-related tasks. This questionnaire presents a Cronbach's alpha of .84 in the original version and .92 in this study.

Hospital Anxiety and Depression Scale

(HADS; Zigmond & Snaith, 1983; Portuguese version of Pais-Ribeiro et al., 2007)

This scale with 14 items consists of two subscales, one that measures anxiety and another depression, each with seven items, answered on an ordinal scale of four points (0 - nonexistent, 3 - very severe), ranging from 0 to 21. The Portuguese adaptation study considers as a cutoff point for anxiety or depression a score equal to or greater than 11. Higher scores indicate greater psychological morbidity. Cronbach's alphas of the

Portuguese version are .76 (anxiety) and .81 (depression). In this study, the total scale was used with an alpha of .90.

Salivettes®

(Sarstedt, Germany) for the collection of saliva and ELISA kits to evaluate salivary cortisol concentrations.

Procedure

This study is cross-sectional and was approved by the Ethics Committee of the Hospitals where the study was carried out. In the hospital group consultations, patients were screened for the inclusion criteria. Subsequently, at the end of the first consultation with the oncologist, participants were approached and those that accepted to participate signed informed consent.

Salivettes, for the collection of saliva to evaluate cortisol, were provided with a leaflet explaining the procedure of use and storage. At the day before the second cycle of chemotherapy, participants collected saliva at about 11pm (the lowest peak of the cortisol pattern) and at the day of chemotherapy shortly after waking up and 30 minutes later. At the day of chemotherapy, the participants delivered the saliva samples and the evaluation protocol was applied, which includes sociodemographic, clinical and psychological measures.

Data Analysis

After evaluating the assumptions for the use of parametric tests, Pearson's Correlation and Point-Biserial tests were performed to evaluate the correlation between sociodemographic, clinical and psychological variables. In order to assess the differences on QoL according to disease stage, a *t* test was performed.

The data were analyzed using the program IBM SPSS® (*Statistical Package for the Social Sciences*), version 25.

RESULTS

Sample Characterization

The sample consisted of 112 participants, aged between 27 and 73 years (*M* = 52.67, *SD* = 10.29) and their disease lasted from 1.5 to 7 months (*M* = 3.96, *SD* = 1.51) receiving the second cycle of chemotherapy. Most women were married and were diagnosed for the first time with BC. Of the total sample, 62% participants were in stage 2. Regarding the number of cycles of prescribed chemotherapy, 36% of women were prescribed 16 cycles, and 33%, 4 cycles. The majority (80%) underwent conservative breast surgery and about 85% of women were taking medication to relieve symptoms (Table 1).

Table 1. Clinical and Sociodemographic Characteristics (N=112)

	n (%)	M (DP)	Min	Max
Age	112	52.67 (10.29)	27	73
Duration of disease (in months)	112	3.96 (1.51)	1.50	7
Marital status				
Single	11 (9.8)			
Married/de facto union	87 (77.7)			
Divorced	8 (7.1)			
Widow	6 (5.4)			
Literary qualifications				
Primary studies	73 (65.2)			
Secondary studies	22 (19.6)			
University	17 (15.2)			
Professional status				
Active worker	4 (3.6)			
Medical Casualty	69 (61.6)			

	n (%)	M (DP)	Min	Max
Unemployed	8 (7.1)			
Reformed	22 (19.6)			
Domestic	9 (8)			
Stage				
Stage 1	43 (38.4)			
Stage 2	69 (61.6)			
Number of cycles				
4 cycles	37 (33)			
6 cycles	24 (21.4)			
8 cycles	11 (9.8)			
16 cycles	40 (35.7)			
Type of surgery				
Breast-conserving Surgery	90 (80.4)			
Mastectomy	7 (6.3)			
Bilateral Mastectomy	2 (1.8)			
Modified Radical Mastectomy	13 (11.6)			

Table 2. Relationship between Sociodemographic, Clinical and Psychological variables

Variables	1	2	3	4	5	6	7	8	9	10	11
1. QOL	-										
2. Age	.064	-									
3. Duration of the disease	.158	.293**	-								
4. Type of surgery (Mastectomy Vs Conservative)	-.160	-.061	-.077	-							
5. Stage (I Vs II)	-.309**	.121	-.113	.134	-						
6. Side effects	-.692***	.071	-.085	.104	.168	-					
7. Psychological morbidity	-.554***	.091	-.063	-.028	.110	.493***	-				

Table 3. (Continued)

Variables	1	2	3	4	5	6	7	8	9	10	11
8. Self-efficacy for coping	.430***	.060	.008	- .116	-.126	-.300**	- .619***	-			
9. Illness perceptions	- .581***	-.040	-.069	.134	.184	.469***	.741***	- .502***	-		
10. CAR	-.250†	-.115	.113	.092	.005	.250	-.108	.081	- .075	-	
11. Cortisol Nadir	.116	-.084	-.081	- .072	- .198*	.121	-.030	.056	- .085	- .102	-

Note. Significance: †$p<.1$, *$p<.05$, **$p<.01$, ***$p<.001$.

Relationship between Sociodemographic, Clinical, Psychological and QoL Variables

Regarding clinical variables, the results showed a negative association between the stage of the disease and QoL as well as between the side effects of systemic therapy and QoL. Thus, more advanced stages of the disease and more side effects resulting from systemic treatment were associated with lower QoL.

Regarding psychological variables, the results revealed a positive association between *coping* and QoL showing that greater self-efficacy in dealing with the tasks associated with cancer were associated with lower QoL. Anxiety, depression, as well as illness perceptions correlated negatively with QoL showing that lower QoL was associated with higher levels of anxiety and depression and a more threatening perception of BC.

The remaining variables (age, duration of disease, type of surgery and nadir cortisol) were not correlated with QoL (Table 2).

Differences in QOL According to Disease Stage

There were significant differences in QoL between patients at stage 1 and patients at stage 2, t (110) = 3.07, p = .003. Patients at stage 1 reported better QoL than patients at stage 2.

DISCUSSION

This study examined the associations between QoL and sociodemographic, clinical and psychological variables in women with BC. The results showed that the disease stage correlated negatively with QoL. In fact, one study also found that QoL was lower as the disease stage increased (Hamer et al., 2016). However, in another study, this association was not found (Gangane, Khairkar, Hurtig, & San Sebastian, 2017). The side effects of systemic therapy correlated negatively with QoL. Effectively, adjuvant chemotherapy treatment has several side effects, such as nausea, vomiting, hair loss, among others, which affect the most patients' daily life (Bushatsky et al., 2017).

Anxiety was also negatively correlated with QoL, as well as depression. There are several studies that corroborate these data (Head et al., 2012; Patoo et al., 2014; Rebholz et al., 2016; Sousa et al., 2015; Tang et al., 2017). In fact, shortly after the diagnosis, patients already present some anxious and depressive symptoms (Høyer et al., 2011) and the same happens at the end of the chemotherapy treatment (Kamińska et al., 2015). Depression and associated symptoms, such as dysphoria, have been associated with less adherence to medical treatment and reduced life expectancy that negatively impact QoL (Reich, Lesur, & Perdrizet-Chevallier, 2008). Depression impacts interpersonal relationships, occupational performance, health perceptions and physical symptoms that, consequently, have an impact on QoL (Somerset, Stout, Miller, & Musselman, 2004) which may explain the results. Also, the undesirable changes in the patient's life due to BC and its treatment are significant sources of anxiety, which, consequently, are associated with worse QoL

(Charalambous, Kaite, Charalambous, Tistsi, & Kouta, 2017). Previous studies have reiterated these findings stating that the changes in women' life due to BC may result in the struggle to achieve a physical and mental self-redefinition that may lead to increased anxiety and lower QoL (Berterö & Wilmoth, 2007).

Self-efficacy for coping was positively associated with QoL. Moradi et al. (2017) also found a significant relationship between coping and the dimensions of QoL including physical health, mental health, social relationships and satisfaction with the environment. The use of more coping strategies may indicate the individual´s attempt to mitigate the loss of activity and independence resulting from the cancer and its treatment, in dealing with physical changes and limitations (e.g., lack of energy, pain, fatigue) in the process of adjusting to a different lifestyle with implications on QoL (Merluzzi et al., 2018).

Perceptions about BC were negatively correlated with QoL, which is corroborated by the literature (Ashley et al., 2015; Kaptein et al., 2015; Tang et al., 2017). In fact, some authors argue that the individual's perceptions of cancer are related to clinical status and behavioral factors, as these can exacerbate the negative symptoms of the disease (e.g., increase in pain) or improve their prognosis (e.g., adherence to treatment) (Figueiras & Marcelino, 2009; Kaptein et al., 2015). Thus, illness perceptions directly influence the individual's emotional response to the disease and its coping behavior (Petrie & Weinman, 2006), affecting QoL (Paek et al., 2016). Therefore, when illness perceptions are negative, patients may present a deeper perception of the symptoms, believing that the disease will last longer and perceiving less control regarding recovery (Petrie & Weinman, 2006). These perceptions, in turn, are associated with inadequate coping strategies, such as non-adherence to treatment (e.g., missing appointments) (Iskandarsyah, Klerk, Suardi, Sadarjoen, & Passchier, 2014) and lower QoL (Puts et al., 2014).

Finally, there were differences in QoL depending on the stage of the disease, as women on stage 1 reported a better QoL than women in stage 2. The literature data resulting from the comparison of QoL of the different stages are inconsistent. In a study by Villar et al. (2017), there were no differences in QoL between different stages (I, II, III, IV). However, in the study by Huang et al. (2013), patients at stage 0 and I revealed a higher QoL than patients in more advanced stages (III and IV). When only stages I and II were compared, no differences were recorded (Tang et al., 2017).

LIMITATIONS AND FUTURE IMPLICATIONS

There are some limitations that must be considered in the present study such as the type of the design that was transversal, not allowing cause and effect relationships to be established, and the fact that most of the instruments were self-report. Also, the majority of patients undergone breast-conserving surgery requiring caution in interpreting the results. Therefore, it would be important, in future studies, to conduct a longitudinal study to evaluate the different phases of the disease with its associated treatments including CAR and analyze their impact over time, on QoL.

CONCLUSION

The results showed that more treatment side effects, a more advanced stage and more negative illness perceptions contributed to a worse QoL, in the second cycle of chemotherapy. Based on these data, BC and chemotherapy, even in the beginning (second cycle) had an impact on QoL. Also, women in stage 2 reported less QoL. It is therefore important, that health professionals take into account the side effects, stage and illness perceptions in designing interventions for women with BC taking also into consideration cortisol levels that are an indicator of stress with implications on coping and adaptation to BC.

REFERENCES

Aaronson, Neil K., Sam Ahmedzai, Bengt Bergman, Monika Bullinger, Ann Cull, Nicole J. Duez, Antonio Filiberti et al. (1993). "The European Organization for Research and Treatment of Cancer QLQ-C30: a quality-of-life instrument for use in international clinical trials in oncology." *JNCI: Journal of the National Cancer Institute* 85(5): 365-376. doi: 10.1093/jnci/85.5.365.

Abercrombie, Heather C., Janine Giese-Davis, Sandra Sephton, Elissa S. Epel, Julie M. Turner-Cobb, and David Spiegel. (2004). "Flattened cortisol rhythms in metastatic breast cancer patients." *Psychoneuroendocrinology* 29(8): 1082-1092.

Armer, Jessica S., Lauren Clevenger, Lauren Z. Davis, Michaela Cuneo, Premal H. Thaker, Michael J. Goodheart, David P. Bender et al. (2018). "Life stress as a risk factor for sustained anxiety and cortisol dysregulation during the first year of survivorship in ovarian cancer." *Cancer* 124(16): 3401-3408. doi:10.1002/cncr.31570.

Ashley, Laura, Joachim Marti, Helen Jones, Galina Velikova, and Penny Wright. (2015). "Illness perceptions within 6 months of cancer diagnosis are an independent prospective predictor of health-related QOL 15 months post-diagnosis." *Psycho-Oncology* 24(11): 1463-1470. doi:10.1002/pon.3812.

Badana, Adrian NS, Victoria R. Marino, Maureen E. Templeman, Susan C. MBCillan, Cindy S. Tofthagen, Brent J. Small, and William E. Haley. (2018). "Understanding the roles of patient symptoms and subjective appraisals in well-being among breast cancer patients." *Supportive Care in Cancer*: 1-8. doi:10.1007/s00520-019-04707-2.

Barsevick, Andrea, Marlene Frost, Aeilko Zwinderman, Per Hall, and Michele Halyard. (2010). "I'm so tired: biological and genetic mechanisms of cancer-related fatigue." *QOL Research* 19, no. 10 (2010): 1419-1427. doi:10.1007/s11136-010-9757-7.

Berger, Ann M., Lynn H. Gerber, and Deborah K. Mayer. (2012). "Cancer-related fatigue: implications for breast cancer survivors." *Cancer* 118(8): 2261-2269. doi:10.1002/cncr.27475.

Berterö, Carina, and Margaret Chamberlain Wilmoth. (2007). "Breast cancer diagnosis and its treatment affecting the self: a meta-synthesis." *Cancer nursing* 30(3): 194-202. doi:10.1097/01.NCC.0000270707. 80037.4c.

Bidstrup, Pernille Envold, Jane Christensen, Birgitte Goldschmidt Mertz, Nina Rottmann, Susanne Oksbjerg Dalton, and Christoffer Johansen. (2015). "Trajectories of distress, anxiety, and depression among women with breast cancer: looking beyond the mean." *Acta Oncologica* 54(5): 789-796. doi:10.3109/0284186X.2014.1002571.

Boing, Leonessa, Camila da Cruz Ramos de Araujo, Gustavo Soares Pereira, Jéssica Moratelli, Magnus Benneti, Adriano Ferreti Borgatto, Anke Bergmann, and Adriana Coutinho de Azevedo Guimarães. (2017). "Tempo sentado, imagem corporal e qualidade de vida em mulheres após a cirurgia do câncer de mama." *Revista Brasileira de Medicina do Esporte* 23(5): 366-370. doi:10.1590/1517-86922017230 5170333. ["Sitting time, body image and quality of life in women after breast cancer surgery." *Brazilian Journal of Sports Medicine*]

Bower, Julienne E., Patricia A. Ganz, Sally S. Dickerson, Laura Petersen, Najib Aziz, and John L. Fahey. (2005). "Diurnal cortisol rhythm and fatigue in breast cancer survivors." *Psychoneuroendocrinology* 30(1): 92-100. doi:10.1016/j.psyneuen.2004.06.003.

Bray, Freddie, Jacques Ferlay, Isabelle Soerjomataram, Rebecca L. Siegel, Lindsey A. Torre, and Ahmedin Jemal. (2018). "Global cancer statistics 2018: GLOBOCAN estimates of incidence and mortality worldwide for 36 cancers in 185 countries." *CA: a cancer journal for clinicians* 68(6): 394-424. doi:10.3322/caac.21492.

Broadbent, Elizabeth, Keith J. Petrie, Jodie Main, and John Weinman. (2006). "The brief illness perception questionnaire." *Journal of psychosomatic research* 60(6): 631-637. doi:10.1016/j.jpsychores. 2005.10.020.

Bushatsky, Magaly, Rafaela Almeida Silva, Maria Theresa Camilo Lima, Mariana Boulitreau Siqueira Campos Barros, João Esberard Vasconcelos Beltrão Neto, and Yasmim Talita de Moraes Ramos. (2017) "Qualidade de vida em mulheres com câncer de mama em tratamento quimioterápico/QOL in women with breast cancer in chemotherapeutic treatment." *Ciência, Cuidado e Saúde* 16(3):1–7. doi:10.4025/cienccuidsaude.v16i3.36094.

Castro, Elisa Kern Kern, Priscila Lawrenz, Fernanda Romeiro, Natália Britz de Lima, and Sílvia Abduch Haas. (2017). "Percepção da Doença e Enfrentamento em Mulheres com Câncer de Mama." *Psicologia: Teoria e Pesquisa* 32(3):1-6. doi:10.1590/0102-3772e32324.

Charalambous, Andreas, Charis P. Kaite, Melanie Charalambous, Theologia Tistsi, and Christiana Kouta. (2017). "The effects on anxiety and QOL of breast cancer patients following completion of the first cycle of chemotherapy." *SAGE open medicine* 5: 1-10. doi:10. 1177/2050312117717507.

Chirico, Andrea, Samantha Serpentini, Thomas Merluzzi, Luca Mallia, Paola Del Bianco, Rosalba Martino, Leonardo Trentin et al. (2017). "Self-efficacy for coping moderates the effects of distress on QOL in palliative cancer care." *Anticancer research* 37(4): 1609-1615. doi:10.21873/anticanres.11491.

Colditz, Graham A., Kimberly A. Kaphingst, Susan E. Hankinson, and Bernard Rosner. (2012). "Family history and risk of breast cancer: nurses' health study." *Breast cancer research and treatment* 133(3): 1097-1104. doi:10.1007/s10549-012-1985-9.

Barros Costa, Victor, Carolina Ribeiro Camargo, Paulo Henrique Fernandes dos Santos, Luciano Ramos de Lima, Marina Morato Stival, and Silvana Schwerz Funghetto. (2017). "Avaliação da qualidade de vida e capacidade funcional de pacientes com câncer em tratamento quimioterápico." *Ciencia, Cuidado e Saude* 16(3): 1–8. doi:10.4025/ cienccuidsaude.v16i3.35663. ["Evaluation of quality of life and functional capacity of cancer patients undergoing chemotherapy." *Science, Care and Health*]

Debess, Jeanne, Jens Østergaard Riis, Lars Pedersen, and Marianne Ewertz. (2009). "Cognitive function and QOL after surgery for early breast cancer in North Jutland, Denmark." *Acta Oncologica* 48(4): 532-540. doi:10.1080/02841860802600755.

Fanakidou, Ioanna, Sofia Zyga, Victoria Alikari, Maria Tsironi, John Stathoulis, and Paraskevi Theofilou. (2018). "Mental health, loneliness, and illness perception outcomes in QOL among young breast cancer patients after mastectomy: the role of breast reconstruction." *QOL Research* 27(2): 539-543. doi:10.1007/s11136-017-1735-x.

Farajzadegan, Ziba, Narjes Khalili, Fariborz Mokarian, and Ali Akbar Morovati. (2015). "Coping skills improve QOL in women with breast cancer and maladaptive coping style." *Social Determinants of Health* 1(1): 18-29. doi:10.1002/pon.3874.

Ferlay, J., M. Colombet, I. Soerjomataram, C. Mathers, D. M. Parkin, M. Piñeros, A. Znaor, and F. Bray. (2018). "Estimating the global cancer incidence and mortality in 2018: GLOBOCAN sources and methods." *International journal of cancer* 144(8): 1941-1953. doi:10.1002/ijc.31937.

Figueiras, Maria João., and Dália Marcelino. (2009). "Exploring associations between illness perceptions and QOL in three chronic illnesses." *Psychology & Health* 24:173-173.

Figueiras, Maria João, Dália Silva Marcelino, Adelaide Claudino, Maria Armanda Cortes, João Maroco, and John Weinman. (2010). "Patients' illness schemata of hypertension: The role of beliefs for the choice of treatment." *Psychology and health* 25(4): 507-517. doi:10.1080/08870440802578961.

Gangane, Nitin, Pravin Khairkar, Anna-Karin Hurtig, and Miguel San Sebastián. "QOL determinants in breast Cancer patients in central rural India. (2017)." *Asian Pacific journal of cancer prevention: APJCP* 18(12): 3325. doi:10.22034/apjcp.2017.18.12.3325.

Gannon, Louisa M., Maura B. Cotter, and Cecily M. Quinn. (2013). "The classification of invasive carcinoma of the breast." *Expert review of anticancer therapy* 13(8): 941-954. doi:10.1586/14737140.2013.820577.

García, Juárez, Dehisy Marisol, René Landero Hernández, Mónica Teresa González Ramírez, and Leticia Jaime Bernal. (2016). "Diurnal cortisol variation and its relationship with stress, optimism and coping strategies in women with breast cancer." *Acta Colombiana de Psicología* 19(1): 113-122. doi:10.14718/ACP.2016.19.1.6.

Garcia, Sabrina Nunes, Carila Galdino, Gisele Cordeiro Castro, Michele Jacowski, Paulo Ricardo Bittencourt Guimarães, and Luciana

Puchalski Kalinke. (2015). "Os domínios afetados na qualidade de vida de mulheres com neoplasia mamária." *Revista Gaúcha de Enfermagem* 36(2): 89-96. doi:10.1590/1983- 1447.2015.02.45718. ["The domains affected in the quality of life of women with breast cancer." *Gaúcha Journal of Nursing*]

Geyikci, Rabia, Soner Cakmak, Mehmet Emin Demirkol, and Sukru Uguz. (2018). "Correlation of Anxiety and Depression Levels with Attitudes Towards Coping with Illness and Sociodemographic Characteristics in Patients with a Diagnosis of Breast Cancer." *Dusunen Adam: Journal of Psychiatry & Neurological Sciences* 31(3):246–257. doi:10.5350/ DAJPN2018310302.

Giese-Davis, Janine, Frank H. Wilhelm, Ansgar Conrad, Heather C. Abercrombie, Sandra Sephton, Maya Yutsis, Eric Neri, C. Barr Taylor, Helena C. Kraemer, and David Spiegel. (2006). "Depression and stress reactivity in metastatic breast cancer." *Psychosomatic medicine* 68(5): 675-683. doi:10.1097/01.psy.0000238216.88515.e5.

Guimarães, Audir Giordano C., and ACY dos Anjos. (2012). "Caracterização sociodemográfica e avaliação da qualidade de vida em mulheres com câncer de mama em tratamento quimioterápico adjuvante." [Sociodemographic characterization and quality of life assessment in women with breast cancer undergoing adjuvant chemotherapy] *Revista Brasileira de Cancerologia* 58(4): 581-92. [*Brazilian Journal of Cancerology*]

Hamer, Julia, Rachel McDonald, Liying Zhang, Sunil Verma, Angela Leahey, Christine Ecclestone, Gillian Bedard et al. (2017). "QOL (QOL) and symptom burden (SB) in patients with breast cancer." *Supportive Care in Cancer* 25(2): 409-419. doi:10.1007/s00520-016-3417-6.

Hayes, Andrew F. 2013. *Introduction to mediation, moderation, and conditional process analysis: A regression-based approach.* New York: Guilford Publications.

Head, Barbara Anderson, Tara J. Schapmire, Cynthia Ellis Keeney, Stacy M. Deck, Jamie L. Studts, Carla P. Hermann, Jennifer A. Scharfenberger, and Mark Paul Pfeifer. (2012). "Use of the Distress Thermometer to discern clinically relevant QOL differences in women with breast cancer." *QOL research* 21(2): 215-223. doi:10.1007/s11136-011-9934-3.

Heitzmann, Carolyn A., Thomas V. Merluzzi, Pascal Jean-Pierre, Joseph A. Roscoe, Kenneth L. Kirsh, and Steven D. Passik. (2011). "Assessing self-efficacy for coping with cancer: development and psychometric analysis of the brief version of the Cancer Behavior Inventory (CBI-B)." *Psycho-Oncology* 20(3): 302-312. doi:10.1002/pon.1735.

Høyer, Marie, Birgitta Johansson, Karin Nordin, Leif Bergkvist, Johan Ahlgren, Annika Lidin-Lindqvist, Mats Lambe, and Claudia Lampic. (2011). "Health-related QOL among women with breast cancer–a population-based study." *Acta oncologica* 50(7): 1015-1026. doi:10.3109/0284186X.2011.577446.

Huang, Rong, Yuan Huang, Ping Tao, H. Li, Qiong Wang, and J. Y. Li. (2013). "Evaluation of the QOL in patients with breast cancer at different TNM stages after standardized treatment." *Zhonghua zhong liu za zhi* [*Chinese journal of oncology*] 35(1): 71-77. doi:10.3760/BCa.j.issn.0253-3766.2013.01.016.

Iskandarsyah, Aulia, Cora de Klerk, Dradjat R. Suardi, Sawitri S. Sadarjoen, and Jan Passchier. (2014). "Consulting a traditional healer and negative illness perceptions are associated with non-adherence to treatment in Indonesian women with breast cancer." *Psycho-Oncology* 23(10): 1118-1124. doi:10.1002/pon.3534.

Jim, Heather S., Michael A. Andrykowski, Pamela N. Munster, and Paul B. Jacobsen. (2007). "Physical symptoms/side effects during breast cancer treatment predict posttreatment distress." *Annals of Behavioral Medicine* 34(2): 200-208. doi:10.1007/BF02872674.

Kaminska, Marzena, Tomasz Ciszewski, Bozena Kukielka-Budny, Tomasz Kubiatowski, Bożena Baczewska, Marta Makara-Studzinska, Elzbieta Staroslawska, and Iwona Bojar. (2015). "Life quality of women with breast cancer after mastectomy or breast conserving therapy treated with adjuvant chemotherapy." *Annals of Agricultural and Environmental Medicine* 22(4):724–730. doi:10.5604/123219661185784.

Kaptein, Adrian A., Kazue Yamaoka, Lucia Snoei, Willem A. Van der Kloot, Kenichi Inoue, T. Tabei, Judith R. Kroep et al. (2013). "Illness perceptions and QOL in Japanese and Dutch women with breast cancer." *Journal of psychosocial oncology* 31(1): 83-102. doi:10.1080/07347332.2012.741092.

Kaptein, Adrian A., Jan W. Schoones, Maarten J. Fischer, Melissa SY Thong, Judith R. Kroep, and Koos JM van der Hoeven. (2015). "Illness perceptions in women with breast cancer—a systematic literature review." *Current breast cancer reports* 7(3): 117-126. doi:10.1007/s12609-015-0187-y.

Kotsopoulos, Joanne, Wendy Y. Chen, Margaret A. Gates, Shelley S. Tworoger, Susan E. Hankinson, and Bernard A. Rosner. (2010). "Risk factors for ductal and lobular breast cancer: results from the nurses' health study." *Breast Cancer Research* 12(6): R106. doi:10.1186/bcr2790.

Lacerda, Gonçalo Forjaz, Scott P. Kelly, Joana Bastos, Clara Castro, Alexandra Mayer, Angela B. Mariotto, and William F. Anderson. (2018). "Breast cancer in Portugal: Temporal trends and age-specific incidence by geographic regions." *Cancer epidemiology* 54: 12-18. doi:10.1016/j.canep.2018.03.003.

Livneh, Hanoch. (2001). "Psychosocial adaptation to chronic illness and disability: A conceptual framework." *Rehabilitation Counseling Bulletin* 44(3): 151-160. doi:10.1177/003435520104400305.

Loo, Wings TY, Michael CW Yip, Louis WC Chow, Qing Liu, Elizabeth LY Ng, Min Wang, and Jianping Chen. (2013). "A pilot study: Application of hemoglobin and cortisol levels, and a memory test to evaluate the QOL of breast cancer patients on chemotherapy." *The International journal of biological markers* 28(4): 348-356. doi:10.5301/JBM.5000053.

Lostaunau, Vanessa, Claudia Torrejón, and Mónica Cassaretto. (2017). "Estrés, afrontamiento y calidad de vida relacionada a la salud en mujeres con cáncer de mama." *Actualidades en Psicología* 31(122): 75-90. doi:10.15517/ap.v31i122.25345. ["Stress, hot flush and quality of life related to health in women with breast cancer." *News in Psychology*]

Ma, Chunhua, Jun Yan, Yan Wu, and Wanbing Huang. (2018). "Illness perceptions of Chinese women with breast cancer and relationships with socio-demographic and clinical characteristics." *International journal of nursing practice* 24(5):1–9. doi:10.1111/ijn.12677.

Matheson, K., & Anisman, H. (2014). In A. W. Kusnecov & H. Anisman (Eds.), *The Wiley-Blackwell Handbook of Psychoneuroimmunology* (pp. 234–250).

Matheson, Kim, and Hymie Anisman. 2014. "Approaches to Assessing Stressor-Induced Cytokine and Endocrine Changes in Humans". In *The Wiley-Blackwell Handbook of Psychoneuroimmunology,* edited by Kusnecov, Alexander W., and Hymie Anisman, 234-250. Oxford: John Wiley & Sons.

Merluzzi, Thomas V., Errol J. Philip, Carolyn A. Heitzmann Ruhf, Haiyan Liu, Miao Yang, and Claire C. Conley. (2018). "Self-efficacy for coping with cancer: Revision of the Cancer Behavior Inventory (Version 3.0)." *Psychological Assessment* 30(4): 486–499. doi: 10.1037/pas0000483.

Moradi, Reza, Mostafa Assar Roudi, Mohammad Mehdi Kiani, Seyed Abdelhossein, Mousavi Rigi, Mahan Mohammadi, Mohammad Keshvari, and Milad Hosseini. (2017). "Investigating the relationship between self-efficacy and QOL in breast cancer patients receiving chemical therapy." *Bali Medical Journal* 6(1):6–11. doi:10.15562/bmj.v6i1.358.

Paek, Min-So, Edward H. Ip, Beverly Levine, and Nancy E. Avis. (2016). "Longitudinal reciprocal relationships between QOL and coping strategies among women with breast cancer." *Annals of Behavioral Medicine* 50(5): 775-783. doi: 10.1007/s12160-016-9803-y.

Pais-Ribeiro, J., Candida Pinto, and Celia Santos. (2008). "Validation study of the portuguese version of the QLC-C30-V. 3." *Psicologia, Saúde e Doenças* 9(1): 89-102. [*Psychology, Health and Diseases*]

Pais-Ribeiro, José, Isabel Silva, Teresa Ferreira, A. Martins, Rute Meneses, and M. Baltar. (2007). "Validation study of a Portuguese version of the Hospital Anxiety and Depression Scale." *Psychology, health & medicine* 12(2): 225-237. doi: 10.1080/13548500500524088.

Patoo, Mozhgan, Ali-Reza Moradi, and Mehrdad Payandeh. (2014). "P0134 Relationship between depression, anxiety, and QOL in women with breast cancer." *European Journal of Cancer* 50(4): e47. doi:10.1016/j.ejca.2014.03.178.

Petrelluzzi, K. F. S., M. C. Garcia, C. A. Petta, D. M. Grassi-Kassisse, and Regina C. Spadari-Bratfisch. (2008). "Salivary cortisol concentrations, stress and QOL in women with endometriosis and chronic pelvic pain." *Stress* 11(5): 390-397. doi:10.1080/10253890701840610.

Petrie, Keith, and John Weinman. (2006). "Why illness perceptions matter." *Clinical Medicine* 6(6): 536-539. doi:10.7861/clinmedicine.6-6-536.

Puts, M. T. E., H. A. Tu, A. Tourangeau, D. Howell, M. Fitch, E. Springall, and S. M. H. Alibhai. (2013). "Factors influencing adherence to cancer treatment in older adults with cancer: a systematic review." *Annals of Oncology* 25(3): 564-577. doi:10.1093/annonc/mdt433.

Rebholz, Whitney N., Elizabeth Cash, Lauren A. Zimmaro, René Bayley-Veloso, Kala Phillips, Chelsea Siwik, Anees B. Chagpar et al. (2018). "Distress and QOL in an ethnically diverse sample awaiting breast cancer surgery." *Journal of health psychology* 23(11): 1438-1451. doi:10.1177/1359105316659916.

Reich, M., A. Lesur, and C. Perdrizet-Chevallier. (2008). "Depression, QOL and breast cancer: a review of the literature." *Breast cancer research and treatment* 110(1): 9-17. doi:10.1007/s10549-007-9706-5.

Rottmann, Nina, Susanne O. Dalton, Jane Christensen, Kirsten Frederiksen, and Christoffer Johansen. "Self-efficacy, adjustment style and well-being in breast cancer patients: a longitudinal study." *QOL Research* 19(6): 827-836. doi:10.1007/s11136-010-9653-1.

Safaee, A., B. Moghimi-Dehkordi, B. Zeighami, H. R. Tabatabaee, and M. A. Pourhoseingholi. (2008). "Predictors of QOL in breast cancer patients under chemotherapy." *Indian Journal of Cancer* 45(3): 107–111. doi:10.4103/0019-509x.44066.

Sapolsky, R. M., & Donnelly, T. M. (2015). Vulnerability to Stress-Induced Tumor Growth Increases with Age in Rats: Role of Glucocorticoids. *Endocrinology, 117*(2), 662–666.

Sapolsky, Robert M., and Thomas M. Donnelly. (1985). "Vulnerability to stress-induced tumor growth increases with age in rats: role of glucocorticoids." *Endocrinology* 117(2): 662-666. doi:10.1016/j.bbi. 2015.10.005.

Schubart, Jane R., Matthew Emerich, Michelle Farnan, J. Stanley Smith, Gordon L. Kauffman, and Rena B. Kass. (2014). "Screening for psychological distress in surgical breast cancer patients." *Annals of surgical oncology* 21(10): 3348-3353. doi:10.1245/s10434-014-3919-8.

Sephton, Sandra E., Robert M. Sapolsky, Helena C. Kraemer, and David Spiegel. (2000). "Diurnal cortisol rhythm as a predictor of breast cancer survival." *Journal of the National Cancer Institute* 92(12): 994-1000. doi:10.1093/jnci/92.12.994.

Sha, Asmin. (2018). "QOL in breast cancer patients–an exploration." *The Breast* 41: S31. doi:10.1016/j.breast.2018.08.090.

Recht, Abram (2016). "Breast Cancer: Stages I-II". *Clinical Radiation Oncology, 1313–1328.e15.* doi:10.1016/b978-0-323-24098-7.00063.

National Institue of Health. 2018. *Breast Cancer.* Acessed July 15. https://report.nih.gov/NIHfactsheets/ViewFactSheet.aspx?csid=73.

Shelby, Rebecca A., Sara N. Edmond, Anava A. Wren, Francis J. Keefe, Jeffrey M. Peppercorn, Paul K. Marcom, Kimberly L. Blackwell, and Gretchen G. Kimmick. (2014). "Self-efficacy for coping with symptoms moderates the relationship between physical symptoms and well-being in breast cancer survivors taking adjuvant endocrine therapy." *Supportive care in cancer* 22(10): 2851-2859. doi: 10.1007/s00520-014-2269-1.

Siegel, Rebecca L., Kimberly D. Miller, and Ahmedin Jemal. (2019). "Cancer statistics, 2019." *CA: a cancer journal for clinicians* 69(1): 7-34. doi:10.3322/caac.21551.

Singletary, S. Eva, Craig Allred, Pandora Ashley, Lawrence W. Bassett, Donald Berry, Kirby I. Bland, Patrick I. Borgen et al. (2003). "Staging system for breast cancer: revisions for the 6th edition of the AJCC Cancer Staging Manual." *Surgical Clinics* 83(4): 803-819. doi:10. 1016/S0039-6109(03)00034-3.

Somerset, Wendy, Steven C. Stout, Andrew H. Miller, and Dominique Musselman. (2004). "Breast cancer and depression." *Oncology (Williston Park, NY)* 18(8): 1021-34.

Sorkhy, Mohammad Al, Zina Fahl, and Jenna Ritchie. (2018). "Cortisol and Breast Cancer: A review of clinical and molecular evidence." *Annals of Cancer Research and Therapy* 26(1): 19-25. doi:10. 4993/acrt.26.19.

Sousa, Helena, Marina Guerra, and Leonor Lencastre. (2015). "Preditores da qualidade de vida numa amostra de mulheres com cancro da mama." *Análise Psicológica* 33(1): 39-53. doi:10.14417/ap.832. ["Predictors of quality of life in a sample of women with breast cancer." *Psychological Analysis*]

Spiga, Francesca, Jamie J. Walker, John R. Terry, and Stafford L. Lightman. (2014). "HPA axis-rhythms." *Comprehensive Physiology* 4(3): 1273-1298. doi:10.1002/cphy.c140003.

Sprangers, M. A., Mogens Groenvold, Juan I. Arraras, Jack Franklin, Adrienne te Velde, Martin Muller, Luisa Franzini et al. (1996). "The European Organization for Research and Treatment of Cancer breast cancer-specific quality-of-life questionnaire module: first results from a three-country field study." *Journal of clinical oncology* 14(10): 2756-2768. doi:10.1200/JCO.1996.14.10.2756.

Steptoe, Andrew., and Bianca, Serwinski. 2016. "Cortisol awakening response." In *Stress: Concepts, cognition, emotion, and behavior*, edited by George Fink, 277-283. Academic Press.

Tang, Lili, Kurt Fritzsche, Rainer Leonhart, Ying Pang, Jinjiang Li, Lili Song, Irmela Fischer et al. (2017). "Emotional distress and dysfunctional illness perception are associated with low mental and physical QOL in Chinese breast cancer patients." *Health and QOL outcomes* 15(1): 1–10. doi:10.1186/s12955-017-0803-9.

Tiezzi, Maria Fernanda Barbirato, Jurandyr Moreira de Andrade, Adriana Peterson Mariano Salata Romão, Daniel Guimarães Tiezzi, Maria Rita Lerri, Hélio Angotti Humberto Carrara, and Lúcia Alves Silva Lara. (2017). "QOL in women with breast cancer treated with or without chemotherapy." *Cancer nursing* 40(2): 108-116. doi:10.1097/ NCC.0000000000000370.

van der Kloot, Willem A., Yuka Uchida, Kenichi Inoue, Kunihiko Kobayashi, Kazue Yamaoka, Hans WR Nortier, and Ad A. Kaptein. (2016). "The effects of illness beliefs and chemotherapy impact on QOL in Japanese and Dutch patients with breast or lung cancer." *Chinese clinical oncology* 5(1). doi:10.3978/j.issn.2304-3865.2016.01.01.

Villar, Raquel Rey, Salvador Pita Fernández, Carmen Cereijo Garea, Mª Pillado, Vanesa Balboa Barreiro, and Cristina González Martín. (2017). "QOL and anxiety in women with breast cancer before and after treatment." *Revista latino-americana de enfermagem* 25. doi:10.1590/1518-8345.2258.2958. [*Latin American Nursing Magazine*]

Wen, Kuang-Yi, and David H. Gustafson. (2004). "Needs assessment for cancer patients and their families." *Health and QOL outcomes* 2(1): 11. doi:10.1186/1477-7525-2-11.

Wöckel, Achim, Lukas Schwentner, M. Krockenberger, Rolf Kreienberg, Wolfgang Janni, Manfred Wischnewsky, Kühn Thorsten et al. (2017). "Predictors of the course of QOL during therapy in women with primary breast cancer." *QOL Research* 26(8),: 2201-2208. doi:10.1007/s11136-017-1570-0.

Zeitzer, Jamie M., Bita Nouriani, Michelle B. Rissling, George W. Sledge, Katherine A. Kaplan, Linn Aasly, Oxana Palesh et al. (2016). "Aberrant nocturnal cortisol and disease progression in women with breast cancer." *Breast cancer research and treatment* 158, no. 1 (2016): 43-50. doi:10.1007/s10549-016-3864-2.

Zigmond, Anthony S., and R. Philip Snaith. (1983). "The hospital anxiety and depression scale." *Acta psychiatrica scandinavica* 67(6): 361-370. doi:10.1111/j.1600-0447.1983.tb09716.x.

Zubrod, Charles G., Marvin Schneiderman, Emil Frei III, Clyde Brindley, G. Lennard Gold, Bruce Shnider, Raul Oviedo et al. (1960). "Appraisal of methods for the study of chemotherapy of cancer in man: comparative therapeutic trial of nitrogen mustard and triethylene thiophosphoramide." *Journal of Chronic Diseases* 11(1): 7-33. doi: 10.1016/0021-9681(60)90137-5.

BIOGRAPHICAL SKETCHES

Inês Pereira

Affiliation: School of Psychology, University of Minho, Braga, Portugal

Education: Master's degree in Psychology

Research and Professional Experience: Member of the Family Health & Illness Research Group

Marta Pereira

Affiliation: School of Psychology, University of Minho, Braga, Portugal

Education: Master's degree in Psychology

Research and Professional Experience: Health Psychology

Publications from the Last 3 Years:

1. Pereira MG, Vilaça M, Pereira M, Bacalhau R, Monteiro S, Fernandes B, … Ferreira G (2019). Validation of the caregiver oncology quality of life questionnaire in Portuguese caregivers of myeloma patients. *Palliative and Supportive Care*, 1–8. DOI: 10.1017/S14789515 19000476.
2. Lopes, A. C., Bacalhau, R., Santos, M., Pereira, M., & Pereira, M. G. (2019). Contribution of Sociodemographic, Clinical, and Psychological Variables to Quality of Life in Women with Cervical Cancer in the Follow-Up Phase. *Journal of Clinical Psychology in Medical Settings*. doi:10.1007/s10880-019-09644-0.
3. Graça Pereira, M., Ferreira, G., Pereira, M., Faria, S., Bacalhau, R., Monteiro, S., … Vilaça, M. (2019). Validation of the Quality of Life Multiple Myeloma Module Questionnaire (QLQ-MY20) in

Portuguese myeloma patients. *European Journal of Cancer Care.* doi:10.1111/ecc.13128.

4. Pereira, M. G., Vilaça, M., Pinheiro, M., Ferreira, G., Pereira, M., Faria, S., ... Bacalhau, R. (2019). Quality of life in caregivers of patients with multiple myeloma. *Aging & Mental Health*, 1–9. doi:10.1080/13607863.2019.1617240.

5. Santos, M., Sousa, C., Pereira, M., & Pereira, M. G. (2019). Quality of Life in Patients with Multiple Sclerosis: A Study with Patients and Caregivers. *Disability and Health Journal*, https://doi.org/10. 1016/j.dhjo.2019.03.007.

6. Pereira, M. G., Machado, J. C., Pereira, M., Lopes, C., & Pedras, S. (2019). Quality of life in elderly Portuguese war veterans with post-traumatic stress symptoms. *Patient Related Outcome Measures,* 10, 49–58. doi:10.2147/prom.s163698.

7. Pereira, M. G., Silva, I., Pereira, M., Faria, S., Silva, B., Monteiro, S., & Ferreira, G. (2018). Unmet needs and quality of life in multiple myeloma patients. *Journal of Health Psychology,* 135910531877207. doi:10.1177/1359105318772073.

8. Pereira, M. G., Roios, E., & Pereira, M. (2017). Functional disability in patients with low back pain: the mediator role of suffering and beliefs about pain control in patients receiving physical and chiropractic treatment. *Brazilian Journal of Physical Therapy,* 21(6), 465–472. doi:10.1016/j.bjpt.2017.06.016.

9. Roios, E., Pereira, M., Machado, J. C., & Pereira, M. G. (2017). Functional Incapacity in Chronic Low Back Pain Patients in Chiropractic versus Physiotherapy Treatment: The Moderator Role of Family Stress. In A. Columbus (ed.), *Advances in Psychology Research* (pp.45-76). Hauppauge, NY: Nova Science Publishers.

10. Teixeira, R. J., Pereira, M., Faria, S., Ferreira, G., & M. Graça Pereira, M. G. (2018). Depression, anxiety and stress levels in adult children caregivers of oncological patients. In R. J. Teixeira, J. Rocha, & V. M. Almeida (Eds.), *Advances in Mental Health Studies* (pp. 4-25). Avid Science ebook.

Ângela Leite

Affiliation: Psychology Research Center (CIPsi), University of Minho, Braga, Portugal

Education: PhD in Psychology (Biomedical Sciences)

Research and Professional Experience: Researcher

Publications from the Last 3 Years:

1. Costa, R., Leite, A., Serra, M. & Sousa, T. (in press). Being psychologically abused is not enough into ending a relationship. *Revista Interamericana de Psicologia. Interamerican Journal of Psychology.*
2. Souto, T., Silva, H., Leite, A., Baptista, A., Queirós, C., & Marques, A. (2019). Facial emotion recognition: VR-REF as a virtual reality trial program for schizophrenic patients. *Rehabilitation Counseling Bulletin.*
3. Leite, A., Dinis, A., Lêdo, S., Gomes, A., & Pinto, A. (2019). Long-term negative psychological impact of presymptomatic testing for Familial Amyloid Polyneuropathy. *Clínica Y Salud.*
4. Leite, A., Ramires, A., Moura, A., Souto, T., & Marôco, J. (in press). Psychological Well-being and Health Perception: Predictors for Past, Present and Future. *Archives of Clinical Psychiatry.*
5. Souto, T., Leite, A., Ramires, A., Santos, V., & Espírito Santo, R. (2018). Perceção da Saúde: validação de uma escala para a população portuguesa. *Trends in Psychology*, 26(4). [Health Perception: validation of a scale for the Portuguese population.]
6. Leite, F., Leite, A., Rasini, BsC, E., Gaiazzi, M., Ribeiro, L., Marino, F., & Cosentino, M. (2018). Dopaminergic pathways in obesity-associated immuno-metabolic depression. *Psychological Medicine*, 1-3. doi.org/10.1017/S0033291718001587.

7. Fernandes, S., McInthyre, T., & Leite, A. (2018). Ajustamento psicossocial ao cancro da mama em função do tipo de cirurgia. *Análise Psicológica*, 36(2), 199-217. doi.org/10.14417/ap.1205. [Psychosocial adjustment to breast cancer according to type of surgery. *Psychological Analysis*]
8. Lêdo, S., Ramires, A., Leite, Â., Dinis, M. A. P., & Sequeiros, J. (2018). Long-term predictors for psychological outcome of pre-symptomatic testing for late-onset neurological diseases. *European Journal of Medical Genetics*. doi.org/10.1016/j.ejmg.2018.03.010.
9. Amorim, S., Leite, Â., & Souto, T. (2017). Sintomatologia depressiva e ansiosa em utilizadores portugueses do Facebook. *Arquivos Brasileiros de Psicologia*, 69(1), 166-183. [Depressive and anxious symptomatology in Portuguese Facebook users. *Brazilian Archives of Psychology*]
10. Dias, D., Leite, A., Ramires, A., & Bicho, P. (2017) Working with cancer: motivation and job satisfaction. *International Journal of Organizational Analysis*, 25 (4), 662-686. doi.org/10.1108/IJOA-12-2016-1096.
11. Lêdo, S., Leite, Â., Souto, T., Pimenta Dinis, M. A., & Sequeiros, J. (2017). Pre-symptomatic testing for neurodegenerative disorders: Middle-to long-term psychopathological impact. *Psicothema*, 29(4). doi.org/10.7334/psicothema2016.298.
12. Leite, A., Leite, F., & Dinis, A. (2017). Subjects at-risk for neurological late-onset genetic diseases: Objective knowledge. *Public Health Genomics*. doi.org/ 10.1159/000479292.
13. Leite, F., Leite, Â., Santos, A., Lima, M., Barbosa, J., Cosentino, M., & Ribeiro, L. (2017). Predictors of subclinical inflammatory obesity: plasma levels of leptin, very low-density lipoprotein cholesterol and CD14 expression of CD16+ monocytes. *Obesity facts*, 10(4), 308-322. doi.org/10.1159/000464294.
14. Dias, D., Leite, Â., Ramires, A., & Bicho, P. (2017). Validação de um instrumento de avaliação dos fatores promotores da motivação para o trabalho: Um estudo com profissionais de saúde oncológica portugueses. *Análise Psicológica*, 35(2), 231-245. doi.org/10.

14417/ap.1255. [Validation of an instrument for assessing factors promoting work motivation: A study with Portuguese cancer health professionals. *Psychological Analysis*]

15. Leite, A., Dinis, A., Sequeiros, J., & Paúl, C. (2017). Risk perception in subjects at-risk for Familial Amyloidotic Polyneuropathy. *Universitas Psychologica*, 16(3). doi.org/10. 11144/javeriana.upsy16-3.rpsf.

16. Leite, F., Leite, Â., & Ribeiro, L. (2017). Blood Donor Characteristics on Transfusion Outcomes—Should Obesity Be Assessed in Future Clinical Trials?. *JAMA internal medicine*, 177(4), 599-599. doi.org/10.1001/jamainternmed.2017.0236.

17. Leite, A., Dinis, A., Sequeiros, J., & Paúl, C. (2017). Motivation to perform presymptomatic testing in portuguese subjects at-risk for late-onset genetic diseases. *Interdisciplinaria*, 34(1), 125-140. doi.org/10.16888/interd.2017.34.1.8.

18. Leite, A., Dinis, A., Lêdo, S., Pinto, A., Gomes, A., & Sousa, H. (2017). Long-term negative psychological impact of presymptomatic testing for Huntington Disease. *Journal of Health, Medicine and Nursing*, 34, 1-9.

19. Reis, P., Leite, A., Amorim, A., & Souto, T. (2016). A solidão em utilizadores Portugueses do Facebook. *Psicologia & Sociedade* 28(2), 237-246. doi.org/10.1590/1807-03102016v28n2p237.

20. Leite, Â., Dinis, M. A. P., Sequeiros, J., & Paúl, C. (2017). Illness representations, knowledge and motivation to perform presymptomatic testing for late-onset genetic diseases. *Psychology Health & Medicine*, 22(2), 244-249. doi.org/10.1080/13548 506.2016.1159704.

21. Lêdo, S., Leite, Â., Souto, T., Dinis, M. A. P., & Sequeiros, J. (2016). Depression as the Middle- and Long-Term Impact for Pre-Symptomatic Testing of Late-Onset Neurodegenerative Disorders. *Trends in Psychology*, 24(2), 579-594. doi.org/10.9788/TP2016.2-11.

22. Lêdo, S., Leite, Â., Souto, T., Dinis, M. A., & Sequeiros, J. (2016). Mid- and long-term anxiety levels associated with presymptomatic

testing of Huntingtons disease, Machado-Joseph disease, and familial amyloid polyneuropathy. *Revista Brasileira de Psiquiatria*, 38(2), 113-120. doi.org/10.1590/1516-4446-2014-1617.

23. Leite, Â., Dinis, M. A. P., Sequeiros, J., & Paúl, C. (2016). Subjects At-Risk for Genetic Diseases in Portugal: Illness Representations. *Journal of Genetic Counseling*, 25(1), 79-89. doi.org/10.1007/s10897-015-9846-4.

M. Graça Pereira

Affiliation: School of Psychology, University of Minho, Braga, Portugal; Psychology Research Center (CIPsi), Braga, Portugal.

Education: PhD in Family Therapy, Florida State University, USA; Aggregation in clinical Research and Health Services, Faculty of Medicine, University of Porto (FMUP)

Research and Professional Experience: University Professor since 1996 in the area of Health Psychology.

Professional Appointments: Associate Professor with Aggregation; Coordinator of the Health Wellbeing, Performance Research Unit; Psychology Research Center (CIPsi). School of Psychology, University of Minho

Honors: 2018 Research Prize, School of Psychology, University of Minho

Publications from the Last 3 Years:

1. Pereira, M. G., Vilaça, M., Pinheiro, M., Ferreira, G., Pereira, M., Faria, S., Monteiro, S., & Bacalhau, R. (in press) Quality of Life in Caregivers of Patients with Multiple Myeloma. *Ageing & Mental Health.*

2. Pereira, M. G., Ferreira, G., Pereira, M., Faria, S., Bacalhau, R., Monteiro, S., Fernandes, B. & Vilaça, M. (in press). Validation of the Quality of Life Multiple Myeloma Module Questionnaire (QLQ-MY20) in Portuguese Myeloma Patients. *European Journal of Cancer Care.*

3. Pereira· M. G., Vilaça, M., Pereira, M., Bacalhau,R., Monteiro, S., Fernandes, B., Faria, S., & Ferreira, G., Vilaça, M., Pereira, M., Faria, S., & Ferreira, G. (*in press*). Validation of the Caregiver Oncology Quality of Life Questionnaire in Portuguese Caregivers of Myeloma Patients. *Palliative & Supportive Care.*

4. Santos, B.D, Carvalho, E. C., & Pereira, M. G. (in press). Dyadic Adjustment in HPV Infected Women One Year After Diagnosis. *Journal of Psychiatry Interpersonal and Biological Processes.*

5. Teixeira, R., Costa-Remondes, S., Brandão, T., & Pereira, M. G. (in press). The impact of informal cancer caregiving: A theoretical study on psychophysiological research. *European Journal of Cancer Care.*

6. Teixeira R., Faria, S., Remondes-Costa, S., Branco, M., Moreira, S., Machado, J. C., & Pereira, M. G. (in press). Brief Emotional Screening in Oncology: Validation of the Emotional Thermometers in the Portuguese Cancer Population. *Palliative and Supportive Care.*

7. Santos, M., Sousa, C., Pereira, M. & Pereira, M. G. (*in press*). Quality of Life in Multiple Sclerosis Patients: A Study with Patients and Caregivers. *Disability and Health Journal.*

8. Santos, D. B., Moreira, C., Vilhena, E., Carvalho, E. & Pereira, M. G. (*in press*). Validation of the HPV Impact Profile (HIP) in Portuguese Women with Human Papilloma Virus. *Current Medical Research & Opinion.*

9. Pereira, M. G., Lopes, H., & Faria, S. (*in press*). Quality of Life One Year after Bariatric Surgery: The Moderator Role of Spirituality. *Obesity Surgery.*

10. Costa· E., Moreira, L., Castanheira, E. & Pereira, M. G. (*in press*). Demographic, Psychological, and Relationship Factors are

Associated with Resource Loss Among Pregnant Women. *Journal of Reproductive and Infant Psychology*.

11. Paredes, A. C., Nabiço, R., Ribeiro, C., & Pereira, M. G. (*in press*). Quality of Life in Breast Cancer Patients: The Moderator Role of Family Stress. *Annals of Psychology*.

12. Pereira, M. G., Pereira, D., & Pedras, S. (*in press*). PTSD, Psychological Morbidity, Marital and Sexual Dissatisfaction in Colonial War Veterans. *Journal of Mental Health*. doi:10. 1080/09638237.2018.1487532.

13. Pucci, S., & Pereira, M. G. (*in press*). The Moderator Role of Caffeine Intake in Adolescents Sleep and Health Behaviors. *Journal of Child and Substance Abuse*.

14. Mata, L., Azevedo, C., Bernardes, M., Chianca, T. Pereira, M Graça, & Carvalho, Emilia. (2019). Efetividade de um programa de ensino para cuidado domiciliar de pacientes prostatectomizados: ensaio clínico controlado randomizado. *Revista da Escola de Enfermagem da USP*, *53*, e03421. doi: 10.1590/s1980-220x 2018012503421. [Effectiveness of a home care teaching program for prostatectomized patients: randomized controlled trial. *USP School of Nursing Journal*]

15. Pedras, S., Preto, I., Carvalho, R., & Pereira, M. G. (2019). Traumatic Stress Symptoms Following a Lower Limb Amputation in Diabetic Patients: A Longitudinal Study. *Psychology & Health*. doi: 0.1080/08870446.2018.1545907.

16. Costa, S., Machado, J. C., & Pereira, M. G. (2018). Burden changes in caregivers of patients with Type 2 Diabetes: A longitudinal study. *Journal of Advanced Nursing*. Epub ahead of print. doi:10.1111/jan.13728.

17. Leite, V., Santos, B. D., & Pereira, M. G. (2018). Psychosocial Impact of Human Papillomavirus on Women's Sexual Dissatisfaction and Quality of Life. *Journal of Psychosomatic Obstetrics & Gynecology*, *3*, 1-7. doi:10.1080/0167482X. 2018.1470164.

18. Mata, L., Bernardes, M., Azevedo, C., Chianca, T., Pereira, M. G., & Carvalho, E. (2018). Método Jacobson e Truax: Avaliação da efetividade clínica de um programa de ensino para cuidado domiciliar pós prostatectomia. *Revista Latino-Americana de Enfermagem*, *26*, e3003. doi:10.1590/1518-8345.2249.3003. [Jacobson and Truax Method: Evaluation of the clinical effectiveness of a teaching program for home care after prostatectomy. *Latin American Journal of Nursing*]

19. Mesquita, A. C., Simão, T. P., Carvalho, A. M., Elias, P. S., Pereira, M. G., & Carvalho, E. C. (2018). The effect of therapeutic listening on anxiety and fear among surgical patients: Randomized Clinical Trial. *Revista Latino-Americana de Enfermagem*, *9*(26). doi:10.1590/1518-8345.2438.3027. [*Latin American Journal of Nursing*]

20. Paredes, C., & Pereira, M. G. (2018). Spirituality, distress and posttraumatic growth in breast cancer patients. *Journal of Religion and Health,* 57(5), 1606-1617. doi:10.1007/s10943-017-0452-7.

21. Pedras, S., Carvalho, R., & Pereira, M. G. (2018). A predictive model of anxiety and depression symptoms after a lower limb amputation. *Disability & Health Journal*, *11*(1), 79-85. doi:10.1016/j.dhjo.2017.03.013.

22. Pedras, S., Vilhena, E., Carvalho, R., & Pereira, M. G. (2018). Psychosocial adjustment to a lower limb amputation ten months after surgery. *Rehabilitation Psychology*, *63*(3), 418-430. doi:10.1037/rep0000189.

23. Pereira, M. G., Pedras, S., & Ferreira, G. (2018). Self-reported adherence to foot care in type 2 diabetes patients: Do illness representations and distress matter? *Primary Health Care Research and Development*, *10*, 1-8. doi:10.1017/S1463423618000531.

24. Pereira, M. G., Pedras, S., Ferreira, G., & Machado, J. C. (2018). Differences, predictors, and moderators of therapeutic adherence in patients recently diagnosed with type 2 diabetes. *Journal of Health Psychology*. Epub ahead of print. doi:10.1177/1359105318780505.

25. Pereira, M. G., Ramos, C., Lobarinhas, A., Machado, J. C., & Pedras, S. (2018). Satisfaction in life with individuals with a lower limb amputation: The importance of active coping and acceptance. *Scandinavian Journal of Psychology, 59*(4), 414-421. doi:10.1111/ sjop.12444 doi: 10.1111/sjop.12444.

26. Pereira, M. G., Silva, I., Pereira, M., Faria, S., Silva, B., Monteiro, S., & Ferreira, G. (2018). Unmet needs and quality of life in multiple myeloma patients. *Journal of Health Psychology.* Epub ahead of print. doi:10.1177/1359105318772073.

27. Romanzini, A., Pereira, M. G., Guilherme, C., Cologna, A. J., & Carvalho, E. C. (2018). Fatores preditores de bem-estar e qualidade de vida em homens submetidos à prostatectomia radical [Predictors of well-being and quality of life in men who underwent radical prostatectomy: longitudinal study]. *Revista Latino-Americana de Enfermagem, 26,* e3031. doi:10.1590/1518-8345. 2601.3031. [*Latin American Journal of Nursing*]

28. Afonso, F., & Pereira, M. G. (2017). Questionário Sociocognitivo para Deixar de Fumar: Construção de um Instrumento baseado na Teoria do Comportamento Planeado. *Revista Iberoamericana de Diagnóstico y Evaluación – e Avaliação Psicológica, 43*(1), 107- 122. doi:10.21865/RIDEP43_107. [Sociocognitive Quiz to Quit Smoking: Building an Instrument Based on the Theory of Planned Behavior. *Ibero-American Journal of Diagnosis and Evaluation - and Psychological Assessment*]

29. Almeida, A., Leandro, E., & Pereira, M. G. (2017). The role of parental illness representations and parental coping in metabolic control of adolescents with Type 1 Diabetes. *Pediatrics and Neonatal Biology, 2*(1), 1-7. Retrieved from.

30. Azevedo, C., Pessalacia, J., Mata, L., Zoboli, E., & Pereira, M. G. (2017). Interface between social support, quality of life and depression in users eligible for palliative care. *Revista da Escola de Enfermagem da USP, 51,* e03245. Epub ahead of print. doi:10.1590/s1980-220x2016038003245. [*USP School of Nursing Journal*]

31. Costa, E., Castanheira, E., Moreira, L., Correia, P., Ribeiro, D., & Pereira, M. G. (2017). Predictors of emotional distress in pregnant women: The mediating role of relationship intimacy. *Journal of Mental Health*, *15*, 1-9. Epub ahead of print. doi:10.1080/09638237.2017.1417545.

32. Costa, E., Castanheira, E., & Pereira, M. G. (2017). Demographic factors, mental health problems and psychosocial resources influence women's AIDS risk. *Health Care for Women International*. Epub ahead of print. doi:10.1080/07399332.2017.1337772.

33. Costa, E, Moreira, L., Castanheira, E., Correira, P., & Pereira, M. G. (2017). Psychological morbidity, social support, and relationship intimacy in pregnant Portuguese women. *International Journal of Pregnancy & Child Birth*, *2*. Ahead-of-print 00040. doi:10.15406/ipcb.2017.02.00040.

34. Costa, S., & Pereira, M. G. (2017). Predictors and moderators of quality of life in caregivers of amputee patients by type 2 diabetes. *Scandinavian Journal of Caring Sciences*. doi:10.1111/scs.12528.

35. Costa, E., Silva, J., & Pereira, M. G. (2017). Demographic factors, mental health problems, and psychosocial resources influence women's AIDS risk. *Health Care for Women International*, *38*(9), 913-926. doi:10.1080/07399332.2017.1337772.

36. Ferreira, G., & Pereira, M. G. (2017). Physical activity: The importance of the extended Theory of Planned Behavior, in type 2 diabetes patients. *Journal of Health Psychology*, *22*(10), 1312-1321. doi:10.1177/1359105315626787.

37. Pedras, S., Carvalho, R., & Pereira, M. G. (2017). A predictive model of anxiety and depression symptoms after limb amputation. *Disability & Health Journal*. Epub ahead of print. doi:10.1016/j.dhjo.2017.03.013.

38. Pereira, M. G. (2017). Changing the mind: Hypnosis and diabetes. *Revista Latino-Americana de Enfermagem*, *25*, e2868. doi:10.1590/1518-8345.0000.2868. [*Latin American Journal of Nursing*]

39. Pereira, M. G., Pedras, S., Ferreira, G., & Machado, J. C. (2017). Family and Couple Variables Regarding Adherence in Type 2 Diabetes Patients in the Initial Stages of the Disease. *Journal of Marital and Family Therapy.* Epub ahead of print. doi:10. 1111/jmft.12281.

40. Pereira, M. G., Ponte, M., Ferreira, G., & Machado, J. C. (2017). Quality of life in patients with skin tumors: the mediator role of body image and social support. *Psycho-Oncology, 26*(6), 815-821. doi:10.1002/pon.4236.

41. Pereira, M. G., Roios, E., & Pereira, M. (2017). Functional disability in patients with low back pain: The mediator role of suffering and beliefs about pain control in patients receiving physical and chiropractic treatment. *Brazilian Journal of Physical Therapy, 21*(6), 465-472. doi:10.1016/j.bjpt.2017.06.016.

42. Roios, E., Paredes, A. C., Alves, A. F., & Pereira, M. G. (2017). Cognitive representations in low back pain in patients receiving chiropractic versus physiotherapy treatment. *Journal of Health Psychology, 22*(8), 1012-1024. doi:10.1177/1359105315621781.

43. Smith, T., Panisch, L. S., Malespin, T., & Pereira, M. G. (2017). Evaluating effectiveness of abstinence education. *Journal of Evidence-Informed Social Work, 14, 360-367.* doi.10.1080/ 23761407.2017.1340860.

44. Teixeira, R., Ferreira, G., & Pereira M. G. (2017). Portuguese validation of the Cognitive and Affective Mindfullness Scale – Revised and the Philadelphia Mindfullness Scale. *Mindfullness & Compassion, 2,* 3-8. doi:10.1016/j.mincom.2017.03.001.

In: Coping with Chronic Illness
Editor: Meghan Mendoza

ISBN: 978-1-53616-775-7
© 2020 Nova Science Publishers, Inc.

Chapter 5

THERAPEUTIC EDUCATION: FROM DISEASE MANAGEMENT TO EMOTION MANAGEMENT

Paola Manfredi[1], and Valentina Turra[2]*

[1]Clinical Psychology, Department of Clinical and Experimental
Sciences, University of Brescia, Italy
[2]ASST Spedali Civili-Brescia, Italy

ABSTRACT

For sometimes, the principles of therapeutic education have been applied to treat adult patients with diabetes. Numerous studies have been conducted in this field, but few have monitored the adherence over time (in "chronicity") of operators and patients.

Although patients are trained in the management of the disease through therapeutic education, over the years the burden of chronicity often hinders the application of principles, skills and known behaviors. It is therefore necessary to monitor coping strategies, the relational dynamics of patients and family members and in particular the management of emotions and resistance to the management of insulin therapy. Furthermore, it is necessary to listen to their emotional and psychological fatigue and anxiety and offer effective help and support

* Corresponding Author's E-mail:paola.manfredi@unibs.it.

strategies. The same is true for health workers, who also suffer from the burden of chronicity.

After reflecting on chronicity, coping strategies, goals of therapeutic education and limits in its implementation, this chapter describes the experience of "continuous" management of adult diabetes at the ASST Spedali Civili of Brescia. The paths dedicated to diabetic patients pay particular attention to the educational-experiential path of Mindfulness, which represents an alternative and appreciated approach based on the recognition of emotions, which is the first filter for their effective management and effective self-care behavior. The results of this pilot study, through the application of BDI, PAID-5 and SCL 90, are disclosed here.

Regarding the management of chronicity by the health team, training and supervision groups have been implemented. In particular, data related to 69 supervisions, 43 medical interviews and 23 nurses based on communication skills and competencies were presented and evaluated.

Clinical work has confirmed that an integrated approach, focused on the recognition of emotions and relational support is a fundamental element in the management of chronicity.

Keywords: therapeutic patient education, mindfulness, coping, supervision, chronic illness, diabetes

1. INTRODUCTION

The trend of the last two decades indicates a constant increase in chronic diseases, which therefore absorb 70% of health costs and represent 80% of the reason for medical consultation.

Among the chronic diseases, the incidence of diabetes has increased insomuch that Wild et al. (2004) speak of a "diabetes epidemic". "The prevalence of diabetes for all age-groups worldwide was estimated to be 2.8% in 2000 and 4.4% in 2030. The total number of people with diabetes is projected to rise from 171 million in 2000 to 366 million in 2030. The urban population in developing countries is projected to double between 2000 and 2030. The most important demographic change to diabetes prevalence across the world appears to be the increase in the proportion of people >65 years of age" (Wild et al. 2004).

"Diabetes mellitus affects more than 12% of the U.S. adult population and has doubled in prevalence between 1990 and 2010. Older adults are particularly affected by the increasing prevalence, which doubles roughly every decade of life and then peaks in the mid-60s at more than 25%." (Andes et al. 2019, p. 1).

According to the American Diabetes Association, about 1.25 million Americans have type 1 diabetes and an estimated 40,000 people will be newly diagnosed each year in the U.S.

Diabetes mellitus is an endocrine pathology; there are different types of diabetes.

Type 1 diabetes (= DM1) usually begins at a young age and is often associated with other autoimmune diseases. The cause of this form of diabetes is a true deficiency of insulin secretion by pancreatic beta cells. Insulin is the hormone that regulates the entry and utilization of glucose by the body. Since pancreatic cells no longer produce this hormone, the body is unable to use circulating glucides (carbohydrates). The glucides failing to enter the cells accumulate in the blood thus causing hyperglycemia, and consequently, the organism metabolizes and burns lipids, to obtain energy instead of glucides, but this leads to the production of ketone bodies as waste metabolites, which are harmful to the body; this phenomenon is known as diabetic ketoacidosis.

Since this disease is irreversible, those affected must take insulin to be able to metabolize sugars. Consequently, patients with type 1 diabetes shall always need daily insulin replacement therapy for the rest of their life.

Type 2 diabetes (= DM2) is usually typical of adults or older people. The cause of this form of diabetes is linked to reduced insulin secretion by pancreatic beta cells also associated with insulin resistance. However, this type of diabetes can appear at any age and sometimes even require insulin therapy. It is frequently found especially in obese subjects.

In both cases, being a chronic disease, care must be constant and daily; control and management of the blood sugar level accompanies the patient with diabetes throughout his life. Many aspects of everyday life must be managed such as food and carbohydrate intake, movement, physical activity and emotions: each of these aspects can cause blood sugar imbalances; therefore, careful monitoring and possible compensation with insulin intake are necessary.

Consequently, diabetes is a chronic condition requiring major attention and intervention by the patient; in fact, diabetes management benefits from a high degree of predictability and routine, but is particularly challenging.

These characteristics make diabetes an elective area for the application of the principles of therapeutic patient education: since diabetes is self-managed, successful care models must focus on strategies that promote and maintain improved self-care behavior (Wolpert, Howard A.; Anderson, Barbara J., 2001).

2. THERAPEUTIC PATIENT EDUCATION

2.1. Therapeutic Patient Education: Principles and Resistances

Therapeutic education (TPE) began in the 1970s, mainly thanks to Jean-Philippe Assal (Lacroix, Assal, 2003) and has long been recognized by the WHO as an effective strategy in the treatment of chronic diseases. "Therapeutic education must enable the patient to acquire and maintain the skills and competencies that help him or her to live optimally with his or her disease. It is, therefore, a permanent process, integrated with care and centered on the patient. Education involves organized awareness-raising activities, information, self-management learning and psychological support in the field of illness, prescribed therapies, therapies, hospital and care facilities, information on the organization and health and illness behaviors. It is designed to help patients and their families understand the illness and its treatment, cooperating with health professionals, living healthier and maintaining or improving their quality of life [...] (Therapeutic education) trains the patient so that he can acquire "knowledge, know-how, ability" to achieve a balance between his everyday life and an optimal control of the disease [...] it is a continuous process that becomes an integral part of the therapy" (1998 WHO). Therapeutic patient education is designed therefore to train patients in the skills of self-managing or adapting treatment to their particular chronic disease, and in coping processes and skills. It should also contribute to reducing the cost of long-term care to patients and society. It is essential to the efficient self-management and to the quality of care of all long-term diseases or conditions, though acutely ill patients should not be excluded from its benefits. Therapeutic patient education is education managed by health care providers trained in the education of patients and designed to enable a patient (or a group of patients and families) to manage the treatment of their condition and prevent avoidable complications while maintaining or improving quality of life. Its principal purpose is to produce a therapeutic effect additional to that of all other interventions (pharmacological, physical therapy, etc.)." (WHO 1998, p. 5).

Therapeutic education is highly effective in all chronic diseases, but it is not at random to think that the widely shared principles that inform therapeutic education have, over time, found rather "hasty" variations.

Lagger, Pataky, Golay (2009) write in their review on the effectiveness of therapeutic education": Il ressort très nettement qu'une très faible proportion des analyses d'études rend compte de la méthodologie de l'éducation thérapeutique mise en place (4%). Le plus souvent, une simple dénomination des cours réalisés est indiquée, par exemple «un ensemble de six séquences didactiques à raison d'une intervention par semaine a été réalisé, par une infirmière, à l'hôpital, concernant le diabète». Les premiers résultats montrent que seulement 27% des études évaluant l'efficacité de l'éducation thérapeutique décrivent correctement la méthodologie."[1]

It is difficult to find, on a theoretical level, arguments contrary to therapeutic education, but, on a practical level, its authentic adoption is not so easy, both for "historical" reasons concerning medical care models, and for the need for investment, time, economic resources, mental (cognitive

---

[1] It is very clear that a very small proportion of study analyses reflect the methodology of therapeutic education implemented (4%). In most cases, a simple name of the courses given is indicated, for example "a set of six didactic sequences at the rate of one intervention per week has been given by a nurse at the hospital concerning diabetes". Initial results show that only 27% of studies evaluating the effectiveness of therapeutic education correctly describe the methodology.

and affective) and creative resources, as well as due to the indispensable and cohesive work team.

Among the historical reasons, it should be recalled that medicine traditionally moves from the perspective of the universal, of invariants, according to a nomothetic and disease-centered approach. This model was adequate and functional as long as the medicine was found to cope with flare-ups, but it is much less so compared to people with chronic illnesses and with fragile patients. The complexity of each patient requires personalized care, for each individual, which is less and less the patient found in the manuals, to which the guidelines apply. Even the same pharmacology explores and pursues individual therapies. Hence the centering on the invariant aspects of diseases and the universal aspects begin to compare with individual perspectives and with a sense of the term "clinical", which was already of a non-modern medicinal origin and is properly linked to clinical psychology. The root of the term "clinical" refers to the Greek etymon κλίνη (read), recalling the original approach that the doctor had with his patient, known in the peculiar characteristics of a sick person, in his context of family, professional and social life, a knowledge that is individualized, longitudinal, built through a relationship (Manfredi, 2018). Moreover, in the past, a medical doctor was the only contact person for the patient and an authority-based relationship was preferred: the patient was asked to comply not to adhere. On the other hand, chronicity requires interdisciplinary work, even better a network, consistent with a bio-psycho-social model, a patient-centered approach; the patient is also asked to play an active, conscious and responsible role.

We can affirm that this general evolution of medicine is perfectly in tune with the spirit of therapeutic education, but its complete realization is in fact still remote. The risk therefore is that therapeutic education can also follow a model that remains prescriptive and based on what the doctor considers correct for the patient. Already in the 1998 WHO report, the need to build a therapeutic education project starting from an analysis of the patient's specificity is emphasized. "Patients with the help of health care providers would define their own learning objectives, in accordance with their life priorities" (p. 17).

More recently Fonte et. al. (2017) highlight "potentially undesirable effects (effects potentially indésirables)"[2] of TPE interventions. In fact, there may be an ideological and normative character in them that patients can experience as a further burden.

We could therefore say that the doctor in the TPE is not only asked to learn but to unlearn: he must unlearn, be able to learn and re-learn!

As the interdisciplinary aspect is inherent in the TPE and is based on the fact that "les individus établissent une mise en relation entre "désordre biologique" et le "désordre scal" pour penser la maladie, cette dernière étant alors représentée comme un état simultanéament biologique et social"[3] (ib, p. 424).

Therapeutic education, therefore, requires a complex structure, a willingness to confront and question. This involves continuous monitoring, which, in our opinion, should not be limited to patients, but, even more importantly, to operators involved through regular team supervision.

If, as far as patients are concerned, questions are raised about the need to have relevant and reliable intermediate result indicators in addition to the specific medical indicators of the disease (Debussche, 2018), the issue regarding the operators is more remote, although it is evident that chronicity is a burden both on patients and operators.

Faced with chronicity, the healthiest answer is creativity, it is an investment surplus. TPE offers ample space in this sense, precisely because the projects must be set in the specificity of the contexts, taking into account the peculiarities of the patients, the operators, the available resources. Among the proposals we can for example recall the "ateliers d'élaboration artistique"[4] (Assal, 2013), le théâtre du vécu (Assal, 2016), the figure of the "collaborative care therapist serving as an outreach health coach for their diabetic patients" (Sieber et al. 2012), video production, integration with telemedicine.

---

[2] potentially adverse effects.
[3] individuals establish a relationship between "biological disorder" and "social disorder" to think of the disease, the latter being represented as a simultaneous biological and social state.
[4] artistic development workshops.

Even when the mental resources for these projects are found, it should not be concealed that economic investment is not irrelevant and this can certainly be another obstacle.

2.2. Therapeutic Patient Education: Coping and Chronic Illness

The demanding investment by the health care team should lead, according to the TPE, to the achievement of an active participation of the patient in his treatment process (Assal, 1996; Barello, 2013).

What is the patient's job? In order to manage one's chronic illness, the patient must take note of the profound and radical change in one's life and self-perception. This change determines the search for a new meaning of oneself, of life, of one's identity. Those who become ill must necessarily and inevitably review their habits, their daily lives, their expectations about the future, their projects; often their role within the family and society changes.

It is undeniable that this process requires significant resources, which are not always available to the extent or in the appropriate quality. Thus, emotional and psychological difficulties can emerge, which often involve the family, the caregivers. It is not uncommon to find that patients have feelings of inadequacy, anxiety related to proving to themselves or others that they can face the demands of the disease, concerns, and anxiety about possible hypoglycemia or hyperglycemia, sadness, and depression for the difficulties incurred in blood sugar management.

Epidemiological investigations have highlighted the high incidence in people with diabetes of disorders such as anxiety, depression, panic disorder, obsessive-compulsive disorder, alexithymia. (Gentili, 2010; Berge, 2015). Poor recognition of these psychopathological problems represents a possible and probable barrier to achieving functional management of emotional problems related to diabetes, with consequent repercussions on the disease itself (Skinner, 2004). In fact, emotions play an important role but prevail in this illness since stress, anger and anxiety can influence glycemia by triggering the axis of the hypothalamic-pituitary-adrenal neuroendocrine system (Nejtek, 2002).

A useful tool for the more functional management of emotions and in general to deal with challenging situations that chronicity may present is represented by coping strategies.

"Coping strategies" mean current cognitive, emotional and behavioral strategies to control specific internal and/or external requests that are evaluated as exceeding the person's resources (Lazarus, 1991). Coping strategies aim at controlling the negative impact of a stressful event, in a dynamic process, where the responses between environment and individual influence one another, in continuous feedback.

Literature, starting from the Endler and Parker's work in 1990, identifies three types of coping principles:

1. task-based coping (task coping), characterized by the tendency to directly tackle the problem, seeking solutions to face the crisis;
2. emotion-focused coping (emotion coping), consisting of specific skills of affective regulation, which allow you to maintain a positive perspective of hope and control of your emotions in a condition of discomfort, or abandonment to emotions, such as the tendency to vent or again, give up;
3. avoidance-based coping (avoidance coping), characterized by the individual's attempt to ignore the threat of the stressful event either through the search for social support or by engaging in activities that divert his attention from the problem. This type of strategy, very often in diabetes management, is counterproductive because people are distracted, try to get rid of the problem and avoid taking care of themselves.

In clinical practice, it is important to recognize and identify which coping strategies can help the patient and his family to cope with diabetes and its chronicity with therapy and life adaptations and readjustments overtime.

It is therefore fundamental to work on the coping strategies that lead the patient to be independent, consistent and effective in managing his therapy.

2.3. Supervision

2.3.1. Centrality of Supervision

A fundamental theme in the management of chronic pathology is the continuous therapeutic education training and supervision of the diabetes team.

Although the subject of discussion is ignored in the literature, in our opinion, the key element for effective therapeutic education is a constant supervision work by the health care team. The main reasons for this need can be seen in some elements characterizing the therapeutic education of the patient, in particular, the quality of the relationship with the patient, the coexistence-combination of different approaches to care, the work carried out in team with various professionals.

2.3.1.1. Relationship with the Patient

Concerning the first topic, as mentioned above, therapeutic education puts the patient at the center of the intervention, but this does not mean that the health care team has a marginal role. On the contrary. Two data can suffice to understand the significance of the effects of the relationships that the caregivers establish with the patients.

In a recent study (Aikens· Piette 2014) it emerged that the degree of nonadherence was significantly associated with the degree to which patients believed that their diabetes medication was unnecessary. However, the patients' perceptions of the necessity and safety of taking medication are primarily transmitted by the caregivers. These are not divergent theoretical interpretations, there are no different schools of thought: the clinical and therapeutic data is clear. What then is the variable at stake? The relationship of trust. The patient can make the doctor's conviction his own only if he considers him a trustworthy person. Faith, unlike an entrustment, needs to be built over time, in the relationship, it is not given *a priori*. The importance of the relationship is also confirmed in the work of Lagger and Golay, which states "The glycemia greatly improved and was strongly correlated with the patient's motivation, the number of training sessions, and the quality of the relationship between the patient and his or her caregiver/instructor."

The skills and interpersonal skills can be learned in training courses, but unlike many other learning mechanisms, a final, definitive point is not reached, there is never the certainty of not making mistakes because every relationship is also a creative act, in which people, we and others, can be new, different, for better or for worse, and previous knowledge, the known schemes can become useless or inapplicable. We may have built good, effective relationships with so many patients, but it is not certain that we will not encounter the situation, the patient or family with whom we will find it difficult to work. In a situation of tension, of non-serenity, the same skills usually employed can be seen as blunt instruments, due to variables ascribable to patients, to the context or to personal aspects of the caregivers who interact in the work situation.

There may be different types of supervision, different ways of "access", more focused on the real interaction with the patient or, as in the Balint groups, on a double side, cognitive and emotional. The latter considered, in particular, both in the operator's countertransference experience in the relationship with the patient and in the relationship between the doctor who reports the case and the Balint group. In the Balint groups, in particular, relational skills are refined, work well-being is promoted, containment of anxieties and frustrations generated by work is offered, new opportunities for interpretation and new ways to approach patients that are perceived as difficult are given. (Balint, 1956).

In addition, a good supervision group also has a narcissistic reinforcement value and can contribute to increasing group cohesion and explicit goal sharing.

2.3.1.2. Coexistence-Combination of Different Treatment Approaches

We have already mentioned how the biomedical paradigm is progressively changing, assuming a perspective of greater centering on the patient; we recall the biopsychosocial patient-centered model, giving greater attention to communication, transition from compliance to adherence (concordance), more stringent legislative indications on informed consent and also a more general epistemological change from classical epistemology to complexity. (Manfredi 2016).

It seems to us, however, that these different perspectives have not found a convincing asset in medicine, but rather give rise to cohabitation, which is sometimes expressed in coherent integrations and others in contradictory forms, in aporia (Manfredi 2012). Without entering into the specifics of this broader discourse, the concept of responsibility for health and care seems to be a crucial element with regard to therapeutic education. Maintaining a balance between doctor and patient is not so obvious, especially since the medical tradition responsibility was seen to be exclusive to the doctor. The difficulty of adopting a different way of thinking finds an emblematic example precisely in the diabetes context, in which, although the standards of care of the American Diabetes Association state that "the management plan should be formulated in collaboration with the patient", the guidelines outline treatment objectives that are formulated entirely from a medical standpoint and focus exclusively on biological endpoints. (Wolpert et al. 2001)

Another indicator of this is the difficulty of involving hospital doctors and the fact that resistance seems to be linked to the feeling of loss of medical power, as well as to the lack of recognition and the belief of a low potential for scientific enhancement of therapeutic education (Rey et al. 2016)

Among the tensions perceived by hospital doctors in the practice of TPE is what is called "tension dialogique", that is the desire for different things, such as between improving the quality of life and physical health, with the feeling of a "derive éducative" (Le Rhun et a. 2013).

Another element that creates discomfort is the affective dimension of the relationship. Here also a certain historical legacy, combined with a reduced formation of relational skills and outdated conceptions of emotions, support the prejudice that the psychologist should handle emotions. Healthcare professionals fear being overwhelmed by the emotions of patients, of not being able to offer answers, of destabilizing people by deepening the knowledge of some events (ib.). But remaining on a purely cognitive level greatly impairs the understanding of the patient and greatly reduces the chances of patient engagement.

2.3.1.3. Different Professional Figures

There are different types of interrelationships among professionals. They are described by various polysemic concepts: multi, inter and transdisciplinary and multi, inter and transprofessionalism. The nature of relationships developed between disciplines is ranged from simple juxtaposition (multidisciplinarity) to integration (transdisciplinarity), through interaction (interdisciplinarity). According to Xavierde la Tribonnière and Rémi Gagnayre (2013), interdisciplinarity is preferred to interprofessionalism due to medical and social disciplines that are shared in a hospital team. Interdisciplinarity offers many benefits but many risks in four areas: project, its building, and deployment, team structure, communication for TPE and training in the field of TPE.

Having different *foci* linked to different professional skills certainly enriches the patient's vision, but on the other hand, there may be discrepancies between the objectives of the professionals and different priorities within the same team.

In addition to the broad themes set out - the relationship with the patient, the co-existence of different approaches to care, the different professional figures -we must also add the availability of resources, to which is also linked a message of greater or lesser consideration of work. In literature, there are more signs for reduced investments and generally the "cuts" or the "supposed savings" intervene more on services for operators than for patients, while we believe that every activity in support of the operators is also for the patients. Consequently, perhaps less discussion regards supervision because only a few centers have invested in this fundamental activity.

3. THERAPEUTIC EDUCATION IN CLINICAL PRACTICE: PRESENTATION OF AN EXPERIENCE

3.1. The Patients

The most advanced health systems, among which the Lombard system, have underlined the necessity to face the problems related to the chronicity cure using new methods in the double sense of territorialization and the ever-closer collaboration in the psycho-social field.

This has involved going from a care model based on services to a model based on the "proactive" and integrated management of the chronic patient. Also, the continuity of hospital-territory assistance aims to accompany the patient, favoring his self-management skills and promoting his well-being.

In this favorable context, there is a project to treat diabetic patients at the ASST Spedali Civili clinic in Brescia.

The key points that have guided and characterize the activity are, consistently with TPE: the attention to the construction of a therapeutic alliance between the patient, his family and the health care personnel, the support of the patient's motivation towards care, the evaluation of his/her resources/readiness to play an active role in the disease management, the outline of a treatment plan that takes into account the need to regulate diet and physical activity based on therapy insulin, assessment and monitoring of the degree of knowledge of the disease itself, assessment of psychosocial factors and psychological screening.

Despite these aspects, not all patients achieve effective disease management; there may be difficulties in the active participation of the patient (Assal, 1991; Barello 2013), in the continuous adherence to treatment, in learning and self-management awareness of the disease. In our experience (Turra, 2016), a frequent obstacle to achieving these goals lies in the psycho-emotional component linked to the disease. In various cases, the role of the psychologist is not always provided for and, if so, he has more of a consultancy than a liaison role. In reality, the effectiveness of this professional is precisely linked to the structural role played on the team, due to its specific role of reflection on the entire project and on the implementation of therapeutic education (Fonte et al. 2017).

At ASST Spedali Civili of Brescia (Italy), thanks to the presence of a psychologist, psychotherapist, on the team, particular emphasis is given to support the patient's psychological well-being, aware of its central role in the course of the disease. In particular, for patients experiencing difficulties in managing type 1 diabetes, a new experimental educational-training offer was developed, also open to family members or caregivers of subjects with diabetes, in order to offer a space for comparison, active sharing between patients and relatives and altogether acquisition of skills and abilities to improve coping strategies, both for the emotional and for the task-centered component.

All the proposed activities follow a cognitive-behavioral approach with the aid of mindfulness. The aim is to integrate the ability to recognize and modify one's cognitive patterns of interpretation regarding experiences and behavioral mechanisms with the ability to center themselves in the present.

Within the therapeutic education pathways, the possibility of individual meetings remains open, particularly at the onset of the disease and upon request of the patient in his chronic condition.

The educational courses within the structure are designed and carried out by the educational group of the team composed of diabetologists, dieticians, and psychologists and reimbursed by the national health system as "group educational therapy". The courses offer different tests of a psychological nature such as the PAID-5 questionnaire (Problem areas in diabetes for stressful diabetes), the ADDQOL (Diabetes Dependent Quality of Life for the evaluation of the quality of life), the BDI (Beck depression inventory for the evaluation of depression), the STAI-Y (State trait anxiety inventory for the evaluation of anxiety), the DTSQ (Diabetes Treatment Satisfaction Questionnaire to assess therapy satisfaction) and SCL-90 (Symptom checklist- 90 for the psychological assessment). The psychological records are inserted into the computerized clinical file, used routinely and viewable by the whole diabetes treatment team, to better integrate the work and the clinical approach between the various operators on the team.

The courses are structured in detail with the division of roles and communication methods to be used based on the different objectives to be achieved.

Among the methodological tools widely used is the "discussion displayed", which uses a methodology used in the world of companies such as meta plan. The group is offered open-ended questions to which each participant responds either verbally or by noting their synthetic thoughts on a card, which is displayed on support visible to all. Contributions are organized, even physically grouping the response cards, thus highlighting some thematic areas. This tool allows the sharing and active participation of all elements of the group both of patients and caregivers and promotes horizontal and non-vertical learning, a learning process that is more accessible and verifiable.

In particular, the proposals are divided into group training and psycho-educational course "intensive insulin therapy management: between strategies and balances not only glycemic", educational-training format: intermediate and final carbohydrate counting, "E-motion between physical activity and emotions" residential course, a formative-experiential group format of Mindfulness.

The various courses are described below. Qualifying elements of the proposal are the Mindfulness group and the supervision by the operators. Some preliminary data is provided below.

Group educational-psychoeducational course "intensive insulin therapy management: between strategies and not only glycemic balances".

This path has been divided into 5 meetings of 3 hours each (from 5 to 8 pm to better accommodate the hourly/working needs of patients) weekly. It includes the combined presence of the doctor, psychologist, and dietitian. The aim is to verify and expand the competences related to the key aspects of intensive insulin therapy (glycemic goals, correction factor, hypo/hyperglycemia, nutrition, carbohydrates, insulin/carbohydrate ratio, physical and sport activity management together with the psychological aspect of emotions. Through the guided discussion/in the training group? Focus group? and the sharing of participants' experiences, the aim is to provide some tools to recognize one's own emotion and understand how this is related to the management of intensive insulin therapy. During the course, the emotions that emerge in the daily diabetes management are explored and the cognitive model of recognition of automatic thoughts and interpretations of reality, the effect of stress on blood sugar, recognition and usefulness even of difficult emotions such as anxiety, fear, anger, sadness, resentment, disgust, shame, and guilt are explained and shared. (Turra, 2016).

Educational-training format: intermediate and final carbohydrate counting.

Group course with a dietician to experiment with carbohydrate counting and alternative measures. The course ends with a day of group work, food management and lunch at the structure.

"E-motion between physical activity and emotions" residential course.

The aim of the course is to transmit competences on the management of intensive and nutritional insulin therapy in people with type 1 diabetes with physical activity. The course is managed by health professionals, doctors, nurses, dieticians, graduates in physical education and is aimed at people with diabetes and their families. It is divided into three residential days. An excursion is an integral part of the itinerary, with mountain guides, on the mountains adjacent to Lake Garda; it is a favorable opportunity to try out the practice of supplements, foods, heart rate monitors, blood glucose and insulin.

It is known that regular physical exercise contributes to an improvement in human health, providing important psychological and physical benefits, particularly at the metabolic, cardiovascular and osteoarticular levels. In patients on intensive insulin therapy, physical activity management requires good preparation, in order to guarantee an efficient and at the same time safe physical performance, avoiding hypo- or hyperglycemia (Lascar, 2014). Work is carried out using the *logbook*, an observational tool on blood sugar levels, nutrition, emotions, and physical activity. The specific setting feeds mutual trust, constant and conscious attention to oneself and others, in a scenario of curiosity, respect and even hilarity (Turra, 2016).

3.1.2. Mindfulness

3.1.2.1. Mindfulness: Educational Strategy and Emotional Coping

With regard to the group paths, a very important space within the structure is also reserved for mindfulness, as a strategy and a tool for the management of chronic illness stress.

Deriving from the Buddhist tradition, in the last 40 years, mindfulness has received increasing attention from the psychological community, especially from cognitive psychology, and from the medical-health community as a means to reduce a significant variety of physical and psychological discomforts ranging from stress, anxiety, depression and chronic pain (Chiesa, 2010, 2011). Jon Kabat-Zinn defines mindfulness as "the awareness that emerges through paying attention on purpose, in the present moment and non-judgmentally, to the unfolding of experience, moment by moment" (Kabat-Zinn, 2003).

Mindfulness is the systematic and intentional development of attention as a whole directed towards current experiences and the adoption of a particular orientation towards experiences in the present moment, characterized by curiosity, openness, and acceptance, without trying to alter or manipulate them in any way (Bishop, 2004). Mindfulness can indicate a *mental state* of conscious and non-judgmental attention to the experience of the present moment, a *trait*, a general attitude present in an individual but variable and *practice*, training with exercises to develop this non-judgmental attention (Chiesa, 2013).

Mindfulness as a practice, strategy, and attitude was introduced in a structured evidence-based protocol (MBSR) in 1979 by Dr. Kabat-Zinn's effort to combine mindfulness-based meditation with clinical and psychological practice, making it suitable to be proposed in a context of modern medicine and western psychology (Kabat-Zinn, 1990). The MBSR program is a protocol of participatory and behavioral medicine with the aim of giving the patient an active role in the awareness and care of himself and his disease. In the following years some scholars and cognitive psychotherapists (Williams, Teasdale, Segal, 2006) developed Mindfulness-Based-Cognitive Therapy (MBCT), a structured path of mindfulness and aspects of cognitive psychotherapy to prevent the relapse into depression, integrating a *body scan, sitting meditation* and *yoga practice or conscious movements* with some aspects of cognitive psychology, such as the cognitive ABC for the recognition of automatic thoughts, the questionnaire of automatic thoughts and other exercises on the awareness of everyday life.

3.1.2.2. Main Scientific Evidence Related to Mindfulness-Based Interventions

Mindfulness-based interventions are to date proven effective for a wide variety of medical and psychological conditions. MBSR appears to significantly reduce physical pain and improve the quality of life in patients suffering from musculoskeletal disorders, fibromyalgia, and rheumatoid arthritis. Evidence shows that MBSR is effective in reducing the emotional load, in terms of stress, hopelessness, anxiety, and depression, in patients with neoplastic diseases or chronic diseases such as diabetes; it could also reduce stress levels in healthcare workers (Chiesa, 2011; Raab, 2014). The MBCT protocol was found to be significantly superior to both placebo and standard treatment for maintenance antidepressant therapy for the prevention of depressive relapse in patients with recurrent major depression. More recent studies have demonstrated the effectiveness of MBSR and MBCT, on the reduction of depression levels in patients with residual depressive symptoms or during a full-blown episode, in numerous anxiety disorders, such as panic attack disorder, the generalized anxiety, social phobia and hypochondria, and substance use disorders (Chiesa, 2011; Keng, 2011). The effectiveness of mindfulness-based protocols has also been confirmed in reducing stress, depressive and anxious symptoms, improving the perception of the quality of life and reducing stress related to management in people with diabetes (Van Son, 2013; Tovote, 2014, Turra, 2018).

Diabetes requires constant attention by the person, focus on tasks, self-checks, and management of the unexpected (food, physical activity, emotions). It is therefore fundamental to learn strategies to remain anchored in the present, to be more centered and to be able to make informed choices and respond to difficulties without reacting impulsively.

3.1.2.3. Educational-Experiential Path of Mindfulness Group (MBSR-Mindfulness-Based Stress Reduction)

Among the range of proposals, the course articulated according to the MBSR protocol - Stressfulness based reduction program (Kabat Zinn, 1990) plays a central and qualifying role. It consists of 8 weekly meetings lasting about 3 hours each (from 5 pm to 8 pm to better accommodate the patients' hourly/working needs) and an intensive day from 10 am to 5 pm. Participants were asked to practice through audio files at least 30 minutes a day of mindfulness meditation at home, and then share and continue the work in the group meeting in the classroom. The ultimate goal of the course is to reduce the levels of stress, anxiety, depression that may be present in a person with diabetes. During this course we share strategies and ways to increase self-awareness through attention and mindfulness meditation exercises; attention is directed to the present with intentionality and a non-judgmental attitude aimed at recognizing and accepting one's thoughts and emotions (Turra, 2016, 2018).

Since 2015, 4 courses have been held for 38 people. Five people did not return the final text of the course, therefore, the analysis sample is composed of 21 females and 12 males, aged between 27 and 63 years with a disease diagnosis from 3 to 40 years. Six SCL 90 protocols were not fully completed and were excluded from the analysis.

The subjects were administered, before and after the course, the BDI (Beck depression inventory) the PAID-5 test (Problem Areas in Diabetes Scale — Five-item Short Form), and SCL 90. - R Symptom Checklist-90-Revised. Despite the quantitative limitation, we can state a clear improvement. In particular, applying the Wilcoxon rank sign test to related samples results in the following statistically significant differences: BDI (p = 000), PAID 5 ((p = 003), SCL 90 global score index (p = 011). also significant are the differences - first - after - in the following SCI subscales: somatization (p = .020), obsession - compulsion (p = .038), depression (p = .009), anxiety ((p = .011), hostility (p = .043).

For further control a parametric test was also applied, normally more robust, although not entirely adequate to the nature of the data. Using the t test for correlated samples, there are significant differences in BDI - t (32) = 6.81, p = .000 - in PAID 5 - t (32) = 2.94, p = .006 - and in the SCL anxiety scale 90 - R - t (26) = 2.05, p = .050.

Obviously, these are preliminary data, but they argue in favor of an investment of this proposal for patients.

3.2. Supervision in Clinical Practice

At the metabolic diabetes division of Internal Medicine at the ASST of the Spedali Civili of Brescia (Italy), a constant training and supervision service has been recently proposed to the team. The objectives are to evaluate and monitor the quality of services, but also to deepen knowledge, through training courses, of the cornerstones of therapeutic education: emotional intelligence, communication, active listening, non-judgment and use of effective communication strategies. For a clinic to function according to the principles of the TPE, everyone (including newly-hired personnel) must know and share goals and objectives. As regards, in particular, the aspect of supervision, the methodology adopted envisages both individual and group work. As regards the first, an assessment is made of the interviews of the health personnel, conducted by the psychologist, according to the observation grids submitted by the team of (J P Assal, 2003). These assessments are then discussed and integrated with the observations of those who conducted the interview. Then there are collective meetings, in which general trends and styles of the department's staff are compared; on the basis of these assessments, the training needs to be strengthened are also outlined.

In particular, the evaluation grid, on a 5-point Likert scale (from 1 for nothing to 5 completely), allows us to focus on some areas. In particular, communication skills and competences were evaluated, with attention to the use of negotiations, the expression of judgments, the use of metaphors, open or closed questions, reformulation. Finally, the conclusion of the interview is evaluated, taking into consideration whether the operator proposes a summary, whether it is responsible to verify the interpretation of the information and whether it delivers the material to the patient, such as the final interview form, the medical applications, medicinal dosages, and upcoming visits.

4. RESULTS

69 supervisions were carried out: 26 nursing and 43 medical. 70% of the observations involved patients with type 2 diabetes, 30% of patients with type 1 diabetes; about 40% of patients were on insulin therapy. The average age was 50 years old.

In 70% of the nursing interviews and in 50% of the medical interviews, negotiation with the patient was observed, a key element of therapeutic education. In 90% of the supervisions, both regarding nurses and doctors, groups, no judgment regarding patients' replies was mentioned. Another important aspect of language and communication is represented by asking closed questions, an aspect that often hinders the expression of the patient: in 68% of the nursing supervisions and in 74% of the medical supervision closed questions were not used. More in detail, the use of closed questions was chosen to facilitate understanding, therefore it was generally used with frail elderly people, characterized by difficulties in understanding the language or cognitive impairment.

Among the other characteristics of communication, a very important aspect is represented by the reformulation by the health worker of what the patient said: this aspect facilitates active listening and creates openness and a sense of understanding for the patient. There is no interview, conducted both by doctors and nurses, in which it is not used. The positive use of the error, i.e., the operator's ability to make the most of the patient's convictions by transforming the methodological, therapeutic errors made by the patient into useful learning mechanisms (prevalence score 3 and 4 on the Likert scale) is also accounted for. Finally, the metaphor is used more in the first interviews, during the initial phase, while it is used less in routine interviews.

In the final part of the educational interventions, the medical and nursing staff summarized what was treated in 75% of the observations and in 90% of the cases the understanding of the patient, passage of absolute relevance, is accounted for.

Another fundamental aspect of the final phase of education/interview is the explanation of the educational and informative material delivered and the sharing of subsequent appointments: this occurred in 80% of cases.

Despite the limited number of the tested subjects and the variability of the clinic type, the data collected shows a good team level in interview management skills. No differences emerge in the two professional groups and this is indicative of shared training. It is important to increase case studies and maintain the team's supervision overtime to preserve quality and attention to educational methods.

The structured supervision activity allowed to highlight the strengths of the team and of each operator and the deficit areas, which can be reinforced in group training courses. By the comparison of both individual operators and the entire healthcare group, the following important topics must be thoroughly examined: assertive communication, open and reflexive listening skills, recognition of emotions and emotional management in education.

CONCLUSION

The clinical progression of diabetes, especially about glycemic control and therapeutic continuity, is largely influenced by the degree of patient involvement in disease management, the success of which depends on a series of psychological, emotional and social factors and the alliance relationship therapy created with the health care team. The therapeutic education approach provides an ideal model for chronicity care, but this approach requires a continuous investment over time, both towards patients and their families and towards operators. The Diabetology Division of

ASST Spedali Civili of Brescia has tried to define the TPE principles by implementing various pathways, with diversified themes and approaches in order to respond to the different needs of patients, who, although all suffering from the same disease, have different characteristics. The data collected, despite the numerical limitations, confirm the effectiveness of this approach.

REFERENCES

Aikens, J. E. & Piette, J. D. (2014). Associations between diabetes patients' medication beliefs and adherence. *Éducation thérapeutique du patient/Therapeutic patient education*, 6(2), 20103. https://doi. org/10.1051/tpe/2014013

AMD, SID. (2018). *Standard Italiani per la cura del diabete mellito.* https://aemmedi.it/wp-content/uploads/2009/06/AMD-Standard-unico1.pdf. [*Italian standards for the treatment of diabetes mellitus.* https://aemmedi.it/wp-content/uploads/2009/06/AMD-Standard-unico1.pdf.].

Andes, L. J., Li, Y., Srinivasan, M., Rolka, D. & Gregg, E. (2019). Diabetes Incidence among Medicare Beneficiaries, 2001-2014. *Diabetes*, Jun, 68 (Supplement 1), 1651. https://doi.org/10.2337/db19-1651-P.

Assal, J. P. (1996). Traitement des maladies de longue durée: de la phase aiguë au stade de chronicité. Une autre gestion de la maladie, un autre processus de prise en charge. *Encyclopédie Médicale Chirurgicale Thérapeutique*, 25-005-A-10. [Treatment of long-term illnesses: from the acute phase to the chronicity stage. Another management of the disease, another process of care. *Therapeutic Surgical Medical Encyclopedia*, 25-005-A-10].

Assal, J. P., Durand, M. & Horn, O. (2016). *Le Théâtre du Vécu. Art, soin, éducation.* Préface de Boris Cyrulnik. Dijon: Raison et passions. [*The Theater of the lived. Art, care, education.* Dijon: Raison et passions].

Assal, T. (2013). L'art et la maladie chronique. Art and chronic illness. *Nutritions & Endocrinologie, 11* (63): 101-106. [Art and chronic illness. *Nutritions & Endocrinologie, 11* (63): 101-106].

Balint, M. (1957). *The doctor, his patient, and the illness.* Oxford: International Universities Press.

Barello, S., Triberti, S., Graffigna, G., Libreri, C., Serino, S., Hibbard, J. & Riva, G. (2016). Health for patient engagement: a systematic review. *Frontiers in Psychology, 6:* 2013.

Beck, A. T., Ward, C. H., Mendelson, M., Mock, J. & Erbaugh, J. (1961). An inventory for measuring depression. *Archives of General Psychiatry, 4:* 561-571.

Berge, L. I. & Riise, T. (2015). Comorbidity between type 2 diabetes and depression in the adult population: directions of the Association and its possible pathophysiological mechanisms. *International Journal of Endocrinology,* 164760. https://doi.org/10.1155/2015/164760.

Bishop, S. R., Lau, M., Shapiro, S., Carlson, L., Anderson, N. D., Carmody, J., Segal, Z. V., Abbey, S., Speca, M., Velting, D. & Devins G. (2004). Mindfulness: a proposed operational definition. *Clinical Psychology, 11*(3): 230-241.

Chiesa A. & Serretti A. (2010). A systematic review of neurobiological and clinical features of mindfulness meditations. *Psychological Medicine, 40*(8): 1239-1252.

Chiesa, A. (2011). *Gli interventi basati sulla Mindfulness. Cosa sono, come agiscono, quando utilizzarli.* Roma: Giovanni Fioriti Editore. [*Interventions based on Mindfulness. What they are, how they act when to use them.* Rome: Giovanni Fioriti Editore].

Chiesa, A. (2013). The Difficulty of Defining Mindfulness: Current Thought and Critical Issues. *Mindfulness, 4*(3): 255-268.

Chiesa, A. & Serretti, A. (2011). Mindfulness-based cognitive therapy for psychiatric disorders: A systematic review and meta-analysis. *Psychiatry Research, 187*(3): 441-53.

Debussche, X. (2018) Le questionnaire heiQ : un outil d'intelligibilité de l'impact de l'éducation thérapeutique dans les maladies chroniques. Analyse dans le cadre de l'investigation d'un programme diabète.

Éducation thérapeutique du patient. *10*(1), 10205. https://doi.org/10.1051/tpe/2018009 [The heiQ questionnaire: assessing the impact of therapeutic education in chronic diseases. The example of a diabetes education program. *Therapeutic patient education, 10*(1), 10205. http://doi.org/ 10.1051/tpe/2018009].

De la Tribonnière, X. & Gagnayr, R. (2013). L'interdisciplinarité en éducation thérapeutique du patient: du concept à une proposition de critères d'évaluation. *Éducation thérapeutique du patient, 5*(1): 163-176. [Interdisciplinarity in patient education: from concept to proposal of evaluation criteria. *Therapeutic patient education, 5*(1): 163-176].

Derogatis, L. R. (1994*). Symptom Checklist-90-R: Administration, scoring & procedure manual for the revised version of the SCL-90.* Minneapolis, MN: National Computer Systems.

Endler, N. S. & Parker, J. D. (1990). Multidimensional assessment of coping: A critical evaluation. *Journal of Personality and Social Psychology, 58*(5): 844-854.

Fonte, D., Lagouanelle-Simeoni. & Apostolidis, T. (2017). Les compétences psychosociales en éducation thérapeutique du patient: des enjeux pour la pratique du psychologue. Psychosocial Skills in Therapeutic Patient Education: Issues for Psychologist Practice. *Pratiques psychologiques.* http://dx.doi.org/10.1016/j.prps.2017.01.005. [Psychosocial Skills in Therapeutic Patient Education: Issues for Psychologist Practice. *Psychological practices.* http://dx.doi.org/10.1016/j.prps.2017.01.005].

Grohmann, B., Espin, S. & Gucciardi E. (2017). Patients' experiences of diabetes education teams integrated into primary care. *Canadian Family Physician. 63*(2): 128-136.

Lacroix, A. & Assal, J. P. (2003). *L'éducation thérapeutique des patients - Accompagner les patients avec une maladie chronique : nouvelles approaches.* 3e édition 2011 Paris: Ed. Maloine. [*Therapeutic Patient Education - Accompanying Patients with Chronic Disease: New Approaches.* 3rd edition 2011 Paris: Ed. Maloine].

Lagger, G., Pataky, Z. & Golay, A. (2009). Efficacité de l'éducation thérapeutique therapeutic. *Revue Médicale Suisse, 5*: 688-690.

[Effectiveness of therapeutic education. *Swiss Medical Journal, 5*: 688-690].

Lagger, G. & Golay, A. (2010). Une éducation thérapeutique en 5 dimensions pour des patients diabétiques de type 1. *Éducation thérapeutique du patient, 2* (2): 117-124. https://doi.org/ 10.1051/tpe/2010013. [A 5-dimensional therapeutic education for type 1 diabetic patients. *Therapeutic patient education, 2* (2): 117-124. https://doi.org/10.1051/tpe/2010013].

Lascar, N., Kennedy, A., Hancock, B., Jenkins, D., Andrews, R. C., Greenfield, S. & Narendran, P. (2014). Attitudes and barriers to exercise in adults with type 1 diabetes (T1DM) and how best to address them: a qualitative study. *PLoS One.* https://doi.org/ 0.1371/journal.pone.0108019.

Lazarus, R. S. (1991). Progress on a cognitive-motivational-relational theory of emotion. *American Psychologist, 46*(8): 819-834.

Le Rhun, A.,Gagnayre, R., Moret, L. & Lombrail, P. (2013). Analyse des tensions perçues par les soignants hospitaliers dans la pratique de l'éducation thérapeutique: implications pour leur supervision. IUHPE – *Global Health Promotion, 20* (2) suppl: 43-47. [Analysis of the tensions perceived by hospital caregivers in the practice of therapeutic education: implications for their supervision. IUHPE – *Global Health Promotion, 20* (2) suppl: 43-47].

Kabat-Zinn, J. (1990). *Full catastrophe living: using the wisdom of your body and mind to face stress, pain and illness.* New York: Dell Publishing.

Kabat-Zinn, J. (2003). Mindfulness-based interventions in context: past, present and future. *Clinical Psychology: Science and Practice*, 10: 144-156.

Keng, S. L., Smoski, M. J. & Robins, C. J. (2011). Effects of mindfulness on psychological health: a review of empirical studies. *Clinical Psychology Review, 31*(6): 1041-56.

Khoury, B., Sharma, M., Rush, S. E. & Fournier, C. (2015). Mindfulness-based stress reduction for healthy individuals: a meta-analysis. *Journal of Psychosomatic Research, 78*: 519-28.

Manfredi, P. (2012). *Parole lievi, parole grevi fra psicologia clinica e medicina*. Roma: Borla. [*Mild words, heavy words between clinical psychology and medicine.* Rome: Borla].

Manfredi, P. (2016). La concordanza nel rapporto medico paziente e la formazione medica. *Medic*, *24*(2): 58-63. [The concordance in the doctor patient relationship and medical education. *Medic*, *24*(2): 58-63].

Manfredi, P. (2018). Aderenza e alleanza: osservazioni psicoanaliche a servizio della medicina. *Recenti Prog Med.*, *109*(4): 226-235. [Adherence and alliance: psychoanalytic observations in the service of medicine. *Recent Prog Med.*, *109* (4): 226-235].

McGuire, B. E., Morrison, T. G., Hermanns, N., Skovlund, S., Eldrup, E., Gagliardino, J., Kokoszka, A., Matthews, D., Pibernik-Okanović, M., Rodríguez-Saldaña, J., de Wit, M. & Snoek, F. J. (2010). Short-form measures of diabetes-related emotional distress: the Problem Areas in Diabetes Scale (PAID)-5 and PAID-1. *Diabetologia*, 53(1): 66-9.

Nejtek, V. A. (2002). High and low emotion events influence emotional stress perceptions and are associated with salivary cortisol response changes in a consecutive stress paradigm. *Psychoneuroendocrinology*, 27: 337-52.

Raab, K. (2014). Mindfulness, Self-Compassion, and Empathy Among Health Care Professionals: A Review of the Literature, *Journal of Health Care Chaplaincy*, 20: 95–108.

Rey, V. & Fontaine, L. (2016). Renforcer l'implication des médecins hospitaliers en éducation thérapeutique: pistes pour la formation continue et l'accompagnement d'équipe. *Éducation thérapeutique du patient*, *8*(1), 10105. https://doi.org/10.1051/tpe/2016005. [Strengthen the involvement of physicians in patient education: tips for training and team's support. *Therapeutic patient education*, *8*(1), 10105. https://doi.org/10.1051/tpe/2016005].

Segal, Z. V., Williams, J. M. G. & Teasdale, J. D. (2006). *Mindfulness-based Cognitive Therapy for Depression*. New York: Guildford Press.

Sieber, W., Newsome, A. & Dustin, L. (2012). Promoting self-management in diabetes: Efficacy of a collaborative care approach. *Families, Systems, & Health, 30*(4): 322-329.

Skinner, T. C. (2004). Psychological barriers. *European Journal of Endocrinology 151*(2): 13-7.

Turra, V., Bonfadini, S., Girelli, A., Zarra, E., Agosti, B., Rocca, L., Cimino, A., Grazioli, G. & Valentini, U. (2016). Percorsi psicoeducativi individuali, di gruppo e di mindfulness nella cura del paziente con diabete di tipo 1. *Giornale italiano di Diabetologia e* Metabolismo, *36*: 50-54. [Individual, group and mindfulness psychoeducational pathways in the care of patients with type 1 diabetes. *Italian Journal of Diabetology and Metabolism*, *36*: 50-54].

Turra V., Bonfadini S., Cimino E., Girelli A. & Valentini U. (2018). Mindfulness: un nuovo strumento per la persona con diabete e per l'operatore sanitario della cronicità. Revisione della letteratura. *JAMD*, 21(2): 93-8. [Mindfulness: a new tool for the person with diabetes and the chronic health worker. Literature review . *JAMD*, *21*(2): 93-8].

Van Son, J., Nyklícek, I., Pop, V. J., Blonk, M. C., Erdtsieck, R. J. & Spooren, P. F. (2013). The effects of a mindfulness-based intervention on emotional distress, quality of life, and HbA(1c) in outpatients with diabetes (DiaMind): a randomized controlled trial. *Diabetes, 36*: 823-30.

Wild, S., Roglic, G., Green, A., Sicree, R. & King. H. (2004). Global prevalence of L.J. *Diabetes Care, 27*(5): 1047-53.

WHO (1998). *Report on Continuing Education programs for Health Care Providers on Therapeutic patient Education in the field of chronic diseases.* http://www.euro.who.int/__data/assets/pdf_file/ 0007/ 145294/E63674.pdf.

Wolpert, H. A. & Anderson, B. J. (2001). Management of diabetes: Are doctors framing the benefits from the wrong perspective? *British Medical Journal, 323*(7319): 994-996.

In: Coping with Chronic Illness
Editor: Meghan Mendoza

ISBN: 978-1-53616-775-7
© 2020 Nova Science Publishers, Inc.

Chapter 6

AGED CARE SERVICES IN THE 'BOOMING' AUSTRALIAN HEALTH CARE INDUSTRY

Peter W. Harvey[1,2,], PhD*
[1]Deakin University, School of Medicine,
Faculty of Health, Geelong, Australia
[2]Flinders University, College of Medicine and Public Health,
Adelaide, Australia

ABSTRACT

A generation ago health care reformers in Australia became interested in managing care for people with chronic conditions to avoid unnecessary hospitalisation for preventable conditions such as diabetes and cardiovascular disease. Indeed, the national coordinated care trials of the late nineties were predicated on these principles and led to the introduction of new primary care management and funding arrangements for Australia, new Medical Benefits Schedule (MBS) item numbers for health assessments, care planning and care coordination along with strategies to train and support the health workforce.

It is now 25 years later, and in my retirement work I am confronted by the enormity of the emerging problem of how to provide good quality,

---

* Corresponding Author's E-mail: peter.harvey@flinders.edu.au, p.harvey@deakin.edu.au, Web: http://www.flinders.edu.au/people/peter.harvey, ORCID: orcid.org/0000-0003-2983-663X.

affordable care and stimulation for an expanding population of older and increasingly dependent people with chronic and complex health needs. This led me to reflect on earlier research work that focused on healthy and productive ageing, care coordination, preventative healthcare and chronic illness management and self-management as strategies for improving health status and reducing hospital admissions for this group of patients.

At the same time, we are regularly reminded of the pressing burden of preventable illness in our younger populations along with our failure as a nation to do anything constructive about reducing obesity and morbidity rates in these groups; the main cause of chronic illness in later life. Whilst we have learnt to manage chronic and complex morbidity better due to the immediate pressures that these illnesses are placing on our acute facilities, we are still not addressing adequately the problem of preventable, lifestyle related illness and morbidity and the lack of health literacy in our community that is adding un-necessary and avoidable pressures to our health care funding and service provision systems.

As our ageing population in Australia is living longer, but with more complex needs, our younger populations are also being impacted prematurely by complex, but essentially preventable health conditions flowing from poor diet, sedentary behaviours and other lifestyle factors. This paper explores options for chronic illness management in aged care facilities while highlighting the need for more effective illness prevention and positive lifestyle management programmes in the earlier years of life.

BACKGROUND

I began driving passenger buses in my retirement, travelling out into metropolitan and rural South Australia, with residents of a large and expanding aged care facility. These community trips helped people remain in touch with the wider elements of society that they tend to become isolated from over time due to their age and reduced mobility. Their resultant experiences prompted me to reflect on some of my related health research work [1-5].

Mostly the residents were extremely grateful for the opportunity to take a trip outside of their care facilities. Many thanked me as if my simple act of driving their bus and helping people to get out and about, along with a bit of chat and the occasional cup of tea or lunch, somehow added value to their lives out of all proportion to my actual input. Community services for aged residents, however, are not the only issue here, and it is evident from the clientele that the needs of these aged care service consumers vary significantly, with some people living with physical and mental disabilities while others show no sign of problems other than their growing inability to function fully in mainstream society due to their age and general physical deterioration.

The current Australian Royal Commission into the aged care sector is exploring how the community might best provide services to cater for the diverse needs of people accessing support from this area of social services [6]. This review explores the question of how, in our currently underfunded health care system, providers might be able to maintain meaningful, high-quality health care services for all residents irrespective of the extent of their frailty, handicap or financial resources? Further, how might it be possible, as in school classrooms for example, to provide a course of study or a set of activities; a regimen of day to day challenges, that takes into account the needs and abilities of all those involved and charts directions for each and every participant for their own unique level of functioning? This would imply that the activities provided should be based on the backgrounds of individual residents, their life experiences, their mental and physical needs and capacities and even their food and physical activity preferences.

INTRODUCTION

In previous generations, the retiree cohort in Australia comprised a relatively small proportion of the overall population. This group did not live long-term into their retirement as a cohort and many people lived with their families or in their own homes in their elderly years. Today the situation is very different with the retired population making up an increasing proportion of the overall Australian population and with more and more ageing Australians living in institutional care. In 2016–17, almost all (97%) people in either type of residential aged care (respite care or permanent residential care) were 65 years of age and over: some

232,000 of these people used permanent residential aged care and some 57,500 used respite residential aged care. In 2017, one in seven Australians (3.8 million) were aged over 65 years of age with 1 in 3 of these people being born overseas, many in non-English speaking counties [7-9]. Projections are that by 2057 around 25% of the Australian population will be aged over 65, with an increasing number of people requiring institutional care of one form or another.

The incidence of chronic and complex illness in this group of ageing Australians is also growing as people live longer and often with multiple chronic conditions (diabetes, COPD, COAD, cardiovascular, musculoskeletal disorders, mental health problems and dementia [10]. The cost to the country's health care system maintaining this ageing population is escalating as are the costs to the individuals who fund their own retirement living arrangements through their savings and superannuation. In addition, at the other end of the continuum, younger people are seen to be developing life-style related chronic illnesses that are essentially preventable. Australia, along with other developed and developing countries [11-15], is therefore facing burgeoning demand in two major age group demographics, the emerging young and the ageing, suggesting that more effective prevention and management of chronic and complex health conditions is the key to managing down the incidence and cost of health care while improving health outcomes across the community [5, 10, 16].

In this context, and whilst we continue to ignore the need for prevention programmes for the young [4], some aged care organisations are building multi-million dollar 'hotel' style apartments to capitalise on an emerging and lucrative market for residents who choose to sell their family homes and move into this style of living while they are still relatively young. Others remain asset rich, but cash poor as they attempt to retain personal independence in their family homes while ageing and as their superannuation funds are depleted over time. It is understandable that the industry would pursue profit where profit options present, but there is a disproportionate effort going into the 'cashed up' parts of the aged care sector at present; the action is where the money is, not where the need is, necessarily. While organisations clamber for the capital and superannuation of the middle class, as a nation we continue to ignore the less well-off people in this sector as well as the health and wellbeing of our younger generations in which preventable chronic illness is creating unnecessary and essentially avoidable morbidity that will compound in older age groups over time [4]. We therefore are seeing escalating demand for health care services at both ends of the demographic in Australia, yet the apparently unprofitable health creation industry we need in the early years of life is being ignored in preference for the more profitable illness industry in the latter years of life [5].

On the positive side, many older people are ageing in healthy and active ways as progressive approaches to ageing in general are promoted in society and older people are encouraged to remain active and continue to participate in and contribute to the wider culture. Older people have much to offer and, if they can maintain their health and wellbeing, are able to remain active and productive members of the community [17-21]. Unfortunately, there are many who, through no fault of their own, do not fit this positive stereotype of healthy and active ageing in Australia.

In this emerging context of health systems change, residents with a wide range of conditions and needs and who are living in aged care facilities and other more intensive care centres are being encouraged, through various activity programmes, to continue to link to and connect with the wider community rather than just existing in their confined living units. Such activities can enhance wellbeing and assist people to manage their complex illnesses better and to live more fulfilling lifestyles [16].

INTERVENTIONS AND SUPPORT OPTIONS

On regular social outings, most residents enjoy the opportunity to chat about various subjects while the odd traveller can be critical of the systems that supports them. This context provides an opportunity for reflection on the national coordinated care initiative that was developed a generation earlier when Australia was setting itself, proactively, to build a preventative health care system focused on community living and service outcomes rather than on hospitals and acute healthcare activity [22-25]. Today, that realty is receding as our reactive health care system struggles, in South Australia in particular, not only to pay for recently constructed hospital infrastructure and to fund the operations of a massive new hospital, but also to cater for the steady growth in the complex health care needs of growing numbers of consumers of health services. The outcomes of this system are fundamentally socially and economically determined [26-28].

Most of the residents living in aged care facilities are extremely grateful for every opportunity they get to expand their horizons and pursue different experiences and daily activities. Like a plane full of locals landing back in Hamburg after a long flight from the antipodes, the aged care residents would often break into spontaneous applause as we neared home base. Unlike the northern dwellers, however, signalling their joy at being back on home ground after a long flight from Singapore or Bangkok I suspect that our local residents tended to celebrate their fleeting respite from, rather than their return to, their familiar safe haven.

In many ways, these centres, their residents and staff embody what the country experienced in its education system in the eighties and nineties; stressed, overworked teachers confronting a disinterested bunch of students, day in day out being offered limited and outdated curricula. There were not enough resources or staff to manage the student learning programmes adequately because each student had different learning needs and functioned at different levels for different subjects while the social changes in society (ie more stressed, overworked and out of their depth parents with no time for their children) and emotional problems of students were becoming more and more problematic. It was a difficult task to teach the students well while attending to other social problems and issues and somehow controlling the mass of students that thronged through the schools each day. It was conjectured, at the time, whether there might ever be enough resources available in schools to ensure that all students reached their educational, social and economic potential [29]. The resource problem still persists today.

The same question is now apt for our ageing population and the operation of the aged care sector. Will there, even with the recent Royal Commission's findings and recommendations, be enough resources committed to this sector to ensure that our elderly people receive dignified, relevant and high-quality care as they live their twilight years in aged care facilities? Could it be that aged care institutions, like our schools, simply replicate the status quo with those who have the personal resources enjoying the best of times while those without resources face the worst of times [30]? Perhaps nothing really changes except the concepts and the language we use to describe what is actually going on over time [31-33].

My experiences of the aged care business also reminded me of papers our teams had published years earlier extolling the virtues of healthy ageing in the context of self-management [5, 10, 16] and the need to ensure that our ageing populations are able to enjoy life while contributing to their society over and above their capacity, simply, to consume and pay for health care and their requisite support services [17]. Even something as simple as offering quality food in these facilities would add value to people's lives; the Maggie Beer Foundation idea, for example [34], along with the self-management concept focused on the needs and goals of individuals being fundamental to the provision of good quality life and care.

AGED CARE ACCOMMODATION RECYCLING

Recently I attended a corporate presentation at an aged care organization to hear that their business was booming and that plans were afoot to move activities interstate and even into other forms of community service provision. The message was, in a nutshell, that the staff were the frontline representatives of a service that put the consumer first. The management team, however, appeared to be much more interested in 'on target' organisational messages than in the day to day reality of the lives of the dependent people for whom they had responsibility for providing good quality care. One member likened a consumer investing their life's savings in a bed in an aged care facility to someone buying a coffee; both the coffee purchaser and the aged care client wanted good service and good value for their money, she insisted, and in a culture of excellence, they would get what they sought.

This is all well and good, but the aged care business model currently turns on the process of recycling the capital of people in need and not on providing a perfunctory coffee en route to the office. Essentially, it goes like this; if residents have a house and superannuation savings, they are a lucrative target of the new iteration of aged care service providers as they shift their business inexorably to focus on privately funded care rather than government supported programmes as retiring people increasingly rely on their self-funded retirement resources rather than on government places in facilities and on the Commonwealth pension for the aged. There is a lot more money in this superannuation pool (6 trillion dollars as of 2018) [35] than ever before and many provider groups are keen to access this resource to fuel and grow their business models while, at the same time, the government is moving to establish new operational guidelines for the sector to underpin quality outcomes for all [36].

Today in Australia, the average retired couple, having worked all their lives and saved their resources, are likely to end up with one or two million dollars, at least, in their house, assets and superannuation, barring major catastrophes along the way. The aged care providers seek to convert this fund pool (family home and superannuation capital) into a package that supports people in their old age. This, at least, is the rhetoric. The reality may be very different. In this new business model, the family home becomes collateral for a bed in a community village, which is fine if the family still owns the capital around such a unit, but many of them do not, and any capital growth occurring over time accrues to the organisations and not to the residents and their families.

The archetypal (perhaps middle class) couple might therefore choose to sell their family home and consolidate their resources to enable them to secure a tiny flat that promises no capital growth potential (at least for the consumer) while the agencies involved make this accommodation available at a fixed rate and then deduct an operating and refurbishment fee from the capital investment of the resident. This means that a million dollars invested today may buy a small unit/home with no capital appreciation for the consumer minus an annual operating and management fee. If a couple lives like this for ten or even twenty years, they would end up with no real estate value to speak of even if their superannuation and health insurance paid for many of their support services in the facility. The family home, over this time, would, therefore, have been sublimated into a tiny asset worth a quarter of its initial value (in real terms) even while the residents' superannuation and or pension funded their day to day accommodation costs and health service requirements along with the standard Medicare component.

So why would people choose to do this? Why would a family sell an asset worth one or two million dollars to buy a tiny unit that with each year that passes would be worth less to its occupants than its purchase value? Private housing accrues capital value (tax free and at least 5% a year, sometimes 10% depending on the town, the suburb and the demand whim) so why should investments in retirement homes be any different? After all, they are investing in houses with capital value that appreciates in markets driven by the principles of supply and demand.

Operating costs should come from a person's superannuation fund, health insurance or pension, but it seems that agencies are also targeting the capital gains on the assets of their clients and residents. As highlighted by the presenter mentioned above, people want value for money; a good service, yet agencies plan to take capital appreciation on housing assets as a component of the cost of living for residents. A unit that costs a half a million dollars in 2019, for example, will command an entry price of three quarters of a million in 2025 for the next generation of consumers, but the original investor stands to see none of this capital growth in real terms. In fact, they and their family will lose considerable capital; losses that compound over time, in addition to day to day costs of living and associated health care services.

The implication is, therefore, that provider agencies will need to position themselves more realistically in the market if they are to continue to attract the substantial resources of the 'baby boomer' generation. Why would a 'baby boomer' forgo their investment growth and trade it for confined accommodation, ordinary food and the odd trip around the block on a sunny day [5, 16]? No. They would want to see capital growth on their investment in real estate accruing to them and to their families over time while their superannuation resource and Medicare benefits funded the support and health services they needed. If this were not the case, surely, they would take their capital in housing, superannuation and investments to a different market. Clearly it is time for the service providers to think beyond the short-term golden egg, especially in relation to the baby boomer generation, which is now the most cashed up and informed group of older consumers, for whatever reason, in Australian history.

If, on the other hand, these facilities offered real value for money, they might be a more attractive proposition to the investor/resident. For example, if in addition to capital security the facility were to maximise patient access to requisite services and care through structured care planning, the package might look more attractive. If the facility were to guarantee high quality input tailored to the needs of individual clients, the package might begin to look more like a viable option for the 'Boomer' generation. Alternatively, they are likely to band together to pool their resources elsewhere while continuing to grow their capital as they have done throughout their lives. They would then be well positioned to buy in the services they needed while continuing to live in their own homes rather than selling up and moving into institutional care where the agency gets the capital gains on property investment and where service provision is linked to MBS resources and private health care cover or a combination of both.

REFERENCES

[1]   Harvey PW. *Coordinated Care and Change Leadership - inside the change process* (research). Perth: University of Western Australia; 2001.

[2]   Harvey PW. Tantalus and the Tyranny of Territory: pursuing the dream of parity in rural and metropolitan population health outcomes

through effective primary health care programmes. Australian *Journal of Primary Health.* 2004;10(3):83-8.

[3]   Harvey PW. Rural Health Systems Change. *Environmental Health.* 2005;5(4):32-40.

[4]   Harvey PW. Social Determinants of Health - why we continue to ignore these factors in the search for improved population health outcomes. *Australian Health Review.* 2006;30(4):419-23.

[5]   Harvey PW. *Self-management and the health care consumer.* Merrick J, editor. New York: Nova Science; 2011. 187 p.

[6]   Harvey PW. The Australian Royal Commission into the aged care industry, 2019. *Journal of Ageing Research and Healthcare.* 2019;2(4):6.

[7]   AIHW. *Older Australia at a glance Canberra*: Australian Institute of Health and Welfare (AIHW); 2018 Available from: https://www. aihw.gov.au/reports/older-people/older-australia-at-a-glance/ contents/demographics-of-older-australians/australia-s-changing-age-gender-profile.

[8]   Commonwealth of Australia. *The Australian Coordinated Care Trials: background and trial descriptions.* Canberra: Commonwealth Department of Health and Aged Care; 1999.

[9]   Menadue J. Final Report of the South Australian Generational Health Review Better Choices Better Health. In: *Health,* editor. Adelaide: South Australian Department of Health; 2003. p. 251.

[10] Battersby MW, Harvey PW, Mills PD, Kalucy E, Pols RG, Frith PA, et al. SA HealthPlus: a controlled trial of a Statewide application of a generic model of chronic illness care. *Milbank Quarterly.* 2007;85(1):37-67.

[11] Chiu TML, Tam KTW, Siu CF, Chau PWP, Battersby M. Validation study of a Chinese version of Partners in Health in Hong Kong (C-PIH HK). *Quality of Life Research.* 2016.

[12] Mei Lee Chiu T, Tai Wo Tam K, Fong Siu C, Wai Ping Chau P. Validation study of a Chinese version of Partners in Health in Hong Kong; C-PIH HK. *Quality of Life Research.* 2015; in process.

[13] Xiaofei Z, Hui F, Lawn S, Mei S, Smith D, Jingxia W, et al. Translation and initial psychometric evaluation of the Chinese version of the partners in health scale. *Biomedical Research.* 2017;28(16):7322-9.

[14] Yu Xu, LiminWang, Jiang He. Prevalence and Control of Diabetes in Chinese Adults. *JAMA.* 2013;310(9):948-58.

[15] Harvey PW. *Chronic condition self-management research planning: a series of lectures.* Centre for Disease Control - invited speaker; October 16-28; Changchun, China 2016.

[16] Harvey PW, Petkov J, Misan G, Warren K, Fuller J, Battersby MW, et al. Self-management support and training for patients with chronic and complex conditions improves health related behaviour and health outcomes. *Australian Health Review.* 2008;32(2):330-8.

[17] Harvey PW, Thurnwald IP. Ageing well, ageing productively – the essential contribution of Australia's ageing population to the social and economic prosperity of the nation. *Health Sociology Review.* 2009;18(4).

[18] Healy J. *The benefits of an ageing population.* The Australia Institute; 2004.

[19] Hugo G, Luszcz M, Carson E, Hinsliff J, Edwards P, Barton C, et al. *State of ageing in South Australia.* Adelaide: SA Government & Office for the Ageing; 2009.

[20] Prime Minister's Science Engineering and Innovation Council. *Promoting healthy ageing in Australia.* Canberra: Department of Health and Ageing; 2003.

[21] *Productivity Commission Research Report.* Economic implications of an ageing Australia. Canberra: Australian Government; 2005. 428 p.

[22] Battersby MW, Harvey PW, Frith P, McDonald P, Kalucy L, Melino M. Health Reform through Coordinated Care: SA HealthPlus. *BMJ.* 2005;330 (March 19):662-5.

[23] Commonwealth of Australia. *The Australian Coordinated Care Trials: Final Technical National Evaluation Report on the First Round of Trials, July 2001.* Canberra: Commonwealth Department of Health and Aged Care; 2001.

[24] Commonwealth of Australia. *Better Health Care - studies in the successful delivery of primary health care services for Aboriginal and Torres Strait Islander Australians.* Canberra: Indigenous and Public Health Media Unit - Commonwealth Department of Health and Aged Care; 2001.

[25] Commonwealth of Australia. The Australian Coordinated Care Trials (COAG)...*Interim National Evaluation Summary.* Canberra: Commonwealth Department of Health and Aged Care; 1999.

[26] Marmot M. Health inequalities among British civil servants: the Whitehall 2 study. *The Lancet.* 1991;337(June):1387-93.

[27] Marmot M. The Solid Facts: The social determinants of health. *Health Promotion Journal of Australia.* 1999;9(2):133-9.

[28] Marmot M, Wilkinson RG. *Social determinants of health.* New York: oxford University Press; 1999. 291 p.

[29] Harvey PW. Distance education and de-schooling. *Dialogue.* 1988;1(2):27-8.

[30] Dickens C. *A tale of two cities.* London1859.

[31] Melville H. *Moby Dick.* London: Collins; 2011.

[32] Hobbes T. Leviathan: or, *The matter, forme & power of a commonwealth, eclesiasticall and civil.* Waller AR, editor. Cambridge: Cambridge University Press; 1651 (1904 Edition).

[33] Marx K, Engels F. *Das Kapital: a critique of political economy* / Karl Marx; edited by Friedrich Engels. Levitsky SL, editor. Chicago: Regnery Gateway; 1952. 356 p.

[34] Beer M. *The Maggie Beer Foundation* 2018 Available from: https://www.maggiebeerfoundation.org.au/.

[35] ABC News. *Paul Keating says raising superannuation to 12 per cent will 'barely cut it: ABC Australia*; 2018 Available from: https://thenewdaily.com.au/money/superannuation/2018/11/14/paul-keating-superannuation/.

[36] Commonwealth of Australia. *Charter of Aged Care Rights 2019* Canberra: Australian Government; 2019 Available from: https://aged care.health.gov.au/quality/single-charter-of-aged-care-rights).

APPENDIX 1. NEW INVESTMENTS IN ACUTE CARE FACILITIES

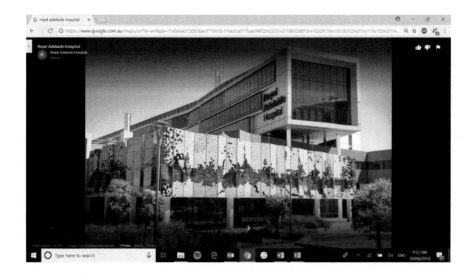

INDEX

D

E

T

U

V

variables, vii, x, 10, 19, 21, 23, 33, 44, 51, 52, 63, 65, 67, 71, 72, 106, 111, 112, 117, 118, 157

W

well-being, vii, ix, 4, 32, 34, 38, 41, 43, 44, 45, 49, 52, 72, 89, 110, 122, 130, 131, 143, 157, 160

workers, xi, 4, 53, 69, 148, 165

workforce, xi, 177

worldwide, 42, 106, 123, 148

worry, vii, ix, 7, 83, 86, 92, 93, 94, 96, 114

Related Nova Publications

IN PURSUIT OF SOCKET HARMONY: OPTIMIZING THE TRANSTIBIAL SOCKET INTERFACE

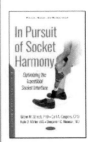

AUTHORS: Glenn M. Street, PhD, Carl A. Caspers, Kyle B. Miller, and Benjamin C. Noonan, MD

SERIES: Physical Medicine and Rehabilitation

BOOK DESCRIPTION: Since the advent of the first modern below-knee prosthesis (joint and lacer) in 1696, the world has seen unprecedented advances in virtually every facet of medical science, yet limb discomfort, pain, and soft tissue breakdown remain a way of life for roughly half of today's ambulatory, below-knee (transtibial) amputees.

HARDCOVER ISBN: 978-1-53615-141-1
RETAIL PRICE: $175

WHEELCHAIRS: PERCEPTIONS, TECHNOLOGY ADVANCES AND BARRIERS

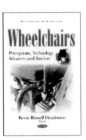

EDITOR: Kevin Russell Henderson

SERIES: Physical Medicine and Rehabilitation

BOOK DESCRIPTION: This book provides new research on the perceptions, barriers and technological advancements of wheelchairs.

SOFTCOVER ISBN: 978-1-53610-390-8
RETAIL PRICE: $82

To see a complete list of Nova publications, please visit our website at www.novapublishers.com

Related Nova Publications

SURFACE ELECTROMYOGRAPHY: FUNDAMENTALS, COMPUTATIONAL TECHNIQUES AND CLINICAL APPLICATIONS

EDITOR: Denise Mitchell

SERIES: Physical Medicine and Rehabilitation

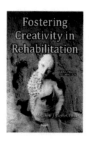

BOOK DESCRIPTION: Surface electromyography (sEMG) represents the electrical activity generated in the muscle fibres in response to the activation provided by the innervation of motor neurons.

HARDCOVER ISBN: 978-1-53610-202-4
RETAIL PRICE: $95

FOSTERING CREATIVITY IN REHABILITATION

EDITOR: Matthew J. Taylor, MD, PhD

SERIES: Physical Medicine and Rehabilitation

BOOK DESCRIPTION: The book begins by examining the emerging science behind individual and organizational creativity, along the way dispelling many myths such as that of the lone genius.

HARDCOVER ISBN: 978-1-63463-259-1
RETAIL PRICE: $215

To see a complete list of Nova publications, please visit our website at www.novapublishers.com